FULL PLATE LESS WEIGHT

HOW TO BE A WEIGHT LOSS WINNER

NEW HOLLAND

For **Jessica** and **Emily**—*my gorgeous daughters who constantly fill my life with inspiration and fill my heart with pride.*

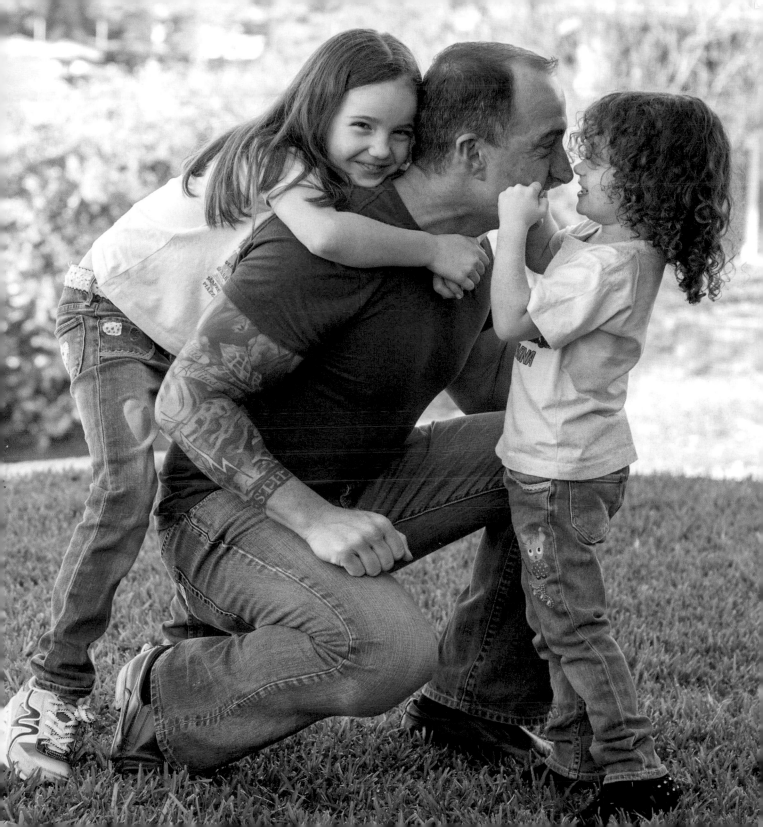

CONTENTS

Acknowledgements

Anyone who has written a book will know that it takes a great deal of work. In the first edition I was blessed enough to have Donna Jones collate all of my information and polish it up into the free-flowing, easy-to-read book it is today. I'd like to thank Donna for the great work she's done in contributing, compiling my information and turning my ideas into reality.

A big special thank you to my family and friends, those who have always been supportive—none of this could have ever happened without you.

And to my many patients past and present, who have helped me further understand the mind and actions of those who struggle day-to-day with the demons of weight loss.

Foreword
A personal note from Johnny Lewis

I first met Ray Kelly on the set of *The Contender*. He would come in each day, putting the fighters through their paces and helping them with their eating plans. Right from the beginning, I could see that this man was different from the rest. He had all the knowledge to engage these high level athletes but, more importantly, he knew how to explain it so they truly understood what they needed to do.

Since that time, I've loved being around Ray and love what he's about. He has helped so many people, not just athletes but those in the community that need it most. His programs on weight loss, diabetes, heart disease, mental health and troubled youth have changed many lives and I believe that the whole country is indebted to him.

There's not a day goes by that Ray isn't helping someone improve their life. It's what he does. It's his gift!

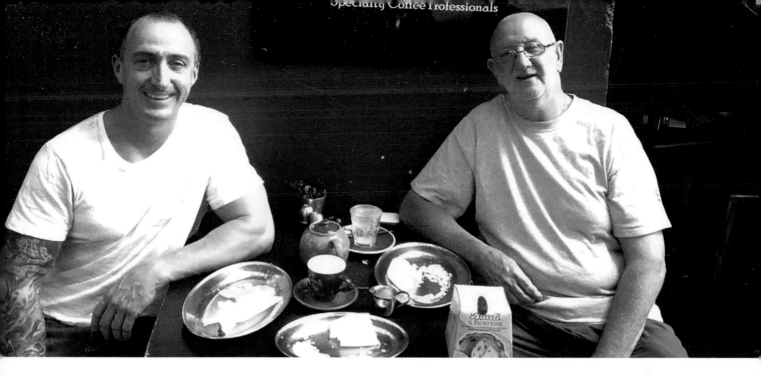

Like me, he was a product of housing commission and it's made him the great person he is today. Ray is a great example of what can be achieved if you really care about others and work hard, no matter where you're starting from. He was always going to be successful because he has nothing but the best motives and lives to help others.

From my own perspective, at 70 years of age, I feel it's important that as you get older you don't just put the cue in the rack. It's very important to believe it's not just over, you need to believe that you still have a part to play in life. We need to fight the health issues that come as we get older and this can mostly be done by walking each day, eating predominantly fresh foods and keeping your mind active. You can't be selfish either; You have to have regular health checks with your doctor.

And it doesn't matter how old you are. It's up to you how you live your life but if you can include some discipline and moderation then you'll be well on your way to a healthy life.

INTRODUCTION

Meet Ray

So who is this guy, you might ask, who trained and coached the two winners of the hit show, *The Biggest Loser*, and helped them grab victory and a whole heap of cash?

I've always been around fitness, having played sport since the age of four, and being heavily into rugby league and rugby union. It wasn't until I had a scrum collapse on me at 19 years old that I injured my lower back and ended up in the gym for rehabilitation—at the time, I had a tiny frame, weighing in at just 60 kilograms (132 pounds). This served as my introduction to a career in health and fitness. Being so scrawny, I had been too intimidated to walk into a gym, as I felt my size would be laughed at by the 'beefy' guys—so I understand how you might feel uncomfortable at the thought of entering a gym full of fit bodies, if you're overweight. After the accident and following need for rehabilitation, it didn't take long for me to become a bit of a 'gym junkie'; I was obsessed with building muscle and got right into the hard-core muscle magazines, supplements, protein powders and rigorous training routines. Aside

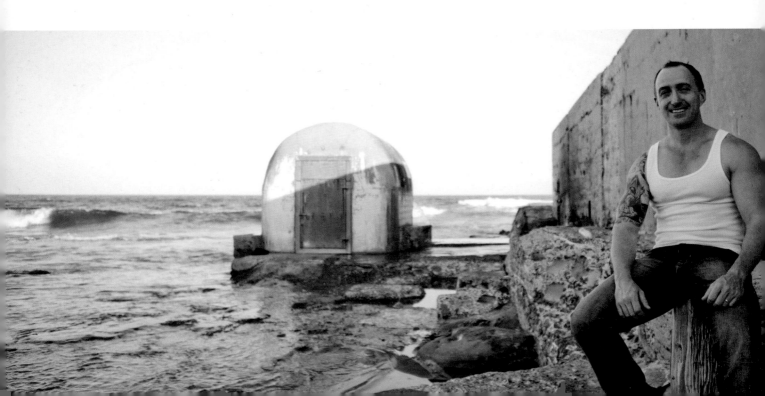

from watching my muscles grow, I started to watch the gym members and the changes they made to their health and fitness, and ultimately their lives. I thought that this was a motivating environment to work in and one where I could make a real difference.

With 15 years in the fitness industry under my belt, my focus gradually turned to weight loss. I realised that a lot of people don't have access to personal trainers and reliable information, and that it was the biggest area that people struggled with. This inspired me to start up a weight loss internet site www.RayKellyFitness.com, which offers support, a chat room and loads of basic and free information for the average person looking to lose weight. I wanted people to be able to ask advice from personal trainers and life coaches, and have a forum where people can share their experiences in an honest and positive way. Today the site has more than 60 000 overweight and obese people who visit each month.

My link to *The Biggest Loser*

Through the site, I got to meet David Hilyander, the first eliminated contestant of the first series of *The Biggest Loser*. After coming out of the house, he stumbled across the site and we chatted online. He happened to be good friends with Adro Sarnelli and told me that Adro had just left the house and that he really needed a trainer. I gave Adro a call and we organised to meet the next day. We started training later that day.

I was quite excited to be involved, as I had watched the US series and was a fan of the show. Adro lived a short five-minute drive from my house, which was perfect for me to train him. In the next seven weeks, I helped him to lose a further 27 kilograms (59 pounds) and take out the title of Australia's first-ever Biggest Loser.

Come the next series the following year Chris Garling had me at the forefront of his mind when he left the house because of my 'winning coach' status. He was very keen to have me work with him—he had told the 'Commando' (boot-camp style personal trainer, who trained two contestants, Chris and Kimberlie Smart, outside of the house before making a surprise entry as 'The Outsiders' in Week 7 of the series) at the very beginning of the series that he was going to contact me when he got out of the house and was hoping that I hadn't already been recruited by one of the other contestants.

I received an email from him two days after he left the house saying that he was eager to train with me and wanted to get things organised ASAP. I gave him a call and we chatted for an hour. My instincts told me right from the start that he had what it takes to give the title a real shake. We organised to meet the following morning at a local coffee shop, started training that day and, with a slightly different training plan to Adro's, seven weeks later it was a case of deja vu: Chris took out the title to become the biggest loser of 2007. And I snatched the title of training back-to-back winners of *The Biggest Loser*.

Why you can become a weight loss winner

Part of the reason why I wanted to write this book is to share with you just what it takes to lose big amounts of weight in short periods of time as Adro and Chris did. They did multiple training sessions a day and ate a very low calorie diet (basically did nothing else other than eat well, train hard and sleep) to lose their weight so quickly. But the biggest reason why I wanted to write this book is to show you that such an extreme approach to weight loss in not only not impractical for most people, but also not necessary to be a successful loser.

You already have all you need to lose weight

'Oh it's easy to lose weight when you're locked in a house, having round-the-clock personal training, calorie-controlled meals and a big wad of cash to spur you on.'

'If I could be confined and earn a weekly wage, I would have the time I need to lose weight without having to worry about the bills because I don't have to work.'

I hear these excuses all the time. You may feel that you have to be isolated to get results but here are your options: You can hold out and hopefully become a contestant on a weight loss TV show (or whatever other excuse you're using for not doing what needs to be done to tackle your weight issues) and put on extra weight in the process—or you can bite the bullet, put your health first and start the process now. Besides, losing weight within the parameters of your own life is much more realistic than being chosen from thousands of applicants to be on a reality weight loss show and being removed from your everyday life in order to lose the weight.

Sooner or later you'll have to deal with everyday food temptations—junk food at every checkout, dinner parties, special occasions, the influence of family members who eat poorly and so on—and everyday time-stealers (usually excuses) that get in the way of exercising, such as work and family commitments. If your diet and exercise routine is restrictive to the extremes, you're not really learning how to behave in the real world. You have to be realistic and practical; not many of us have unlimited time to do multiple training sessions and prepare a strict diet. So the sooner you learn how to lose weight within your everyday life, the better. And this book shows you how.

Why will my approach work?

Why trust me over another? It's confusing out there with so many weight loss solutions on offer, but mine is based on facts, and you only need to look at the success Chris and Adro experienced as the evidence. I had no secret training method or special diet for Chris and Adro; just a calorie-controlled eating plan and a lot of hard work in the exercise department!

My program is very progressive—it's not just slapped together. A lot of thought has gone into each training session and into what works best on what day to guarantee results. You just have to back yourself and give it a go!

So, what's been happening since the last edition?

Since the first edition, so much has happened in both my personal and business life, teaching me quite a lot about weight loss and life in general. So it seemed essential that I provide an updated version of this book.

Firstly, and most importantly, I was blessed with another daughter, Emily. I'm sure all parents would agree that it's great to watch each child turn into their own little person. While parenting can seem complex at times, I do believe it makes life simpler too. Being a parent is a great responsibility; no doubt the greatest of our life and it is something I do not take lightly. My choices and actions (both health related and otherwise) will have a major impact on the beliefs of my children, and in turn their children as well. While it may not be easy initially, if I ensure my children are reasonably active and eat mostly fresh foods there is a great chance that they will not suffer many of the conditions found in many adults today. They may not have to worry about type 2 diabetes, hypertension and cholesterol medications in their 30's. In fact, they may just end up being an active parent with their children too.

It may not be easy but what other choice do you have? To help you along I've outlined a simple children's meal plan to get you started. My girls have also provided some tips of their own on page 207!

As I wrote in the last edition I've had a strong background in sport, preparing athletes for Olympic Games and world championship competition. I made a return to the sporting arena working with many world-class professional fighters in the disciplines of boxing, kickboxing, and mixed martial arts. In fact, since 2008, I've worked with more than 10 world champions. In addition to that, I was employed as a consultant on the boxing reality TV show *The Contender*, and even got to work the corner for a world title fight at the MGM Grand in Las Vegas.

Ongoing education has also been a primary focus for me. I've graduated with a Masters in Teaching, and travelled the world attending conferences on obesity and metabolic diseases. At these conferences I was able to discuss my program with the presenters and receive feedback from some of the smartest people involved in weight loss research. I've incorporated many new research based ideas in my clinics, with sensational results for my patients, both on the scales and metabolically.

So here you have it! The updated version of my book. Put these methods into practice and I can promise you the same kind of transformation I have been providing my patients with over the last 22 years!

What I've learnt since the last edition

- We know enough about weight loss itself to change the lives of most obese people. The issue is: how do we change behaviour? This is where I believe more research should be targeted.

- Meal replacement shakes, like surgery, have a role to play in weight loss. With shakes, make sure the product you buy has a solid eating and exercise plan behind it and is prescribed by a suitably qualified professional. If you are considering surgery, look at all other avenues first. If you are under 120 kg and can't lose weight by changing your lifestyle there is little chance surgery will work for you either. Even with surgery you need to change your lifestyle.

- Fast weight loss is a very safe and effective way to lose weight if it is done correctly. The research is out and positive results are building.

- Type 2 diabetics should not be given carbohydrates with every meal. Body fat loss should be the first treatment for Type 2 diabetes and this is done faster and easier when reducing carbohydrates. They can then be added back in progressively as the patient gets closer to goal weight, and can process them much more efficiently.

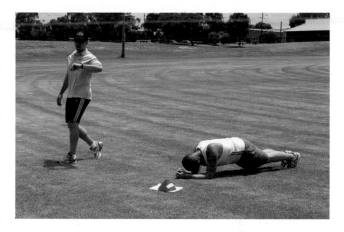

- Women with Polycystic Ovarian Syndrome (PCOS) don't actually lose weight slower than those that don't have the condition. I was always taught that these women lose weight slower but have since found that the issue for many is that they have also become insulin resistant. When treated as a type 2 diabetic they often lose weight just as easily as those that don't suffer from PCOS.

- There is nothing more important than your health. Without good health you have nothing.

- You don't have to be thin to be healthy. Keep your BMI under 30, walk every day and eat predominantly fresh foods and you should be fine.

- The medical profession will keep us alive much longer, but our quality of life may be just as poor for over half of our life if we don't take control of our health. Many health conditions can be traced back to lifestyle, from Type 2 diabetes, heart disease and, in some cases, depression.

- Face your fears! How do you know how great you might be if you don't try?

- You will die, so why not make the most of every minute you have on this earth?

A final word

I believe that everyone can lose weight, no matter where you're at, how many false starts you've had, or what obstacles are standing in your way. Because you're always learning each time you try. You've got a different set of circumstances each time, which contain a different set of lessons. You've only failed if you haven't taken anything away from your previous attempts to lose weight. Each time you try, if you implement what you have learnt, you will get better and better at it. Slowly, but surely, you will learn the tricks and be successful.

To lose weight you have to keep putting one foot in front of the other. When you slip up—and you will because everyone does and none of us are perfect—you can't let it get you down. You just have to learn from the experience and keep moving forward. If you can walk, you can do it. You don't need money for trainers, gyms or complicated diets. There's no doubt that you may find it hard at the start, but I can absolutely promise you that it gets much easier. You can tell yourself all sorts of lies but I know what you're capable of. I won't let you quit. Perseverance is the most important component of weight loss.

Just give me your commitment and I can help you turn things around.

How to use this book

Each part of this book will walk you through the diet and exercise changes you need to make to become a successful weight loss winner. The book will walk you through the steps necessary to achieve success at a rate that suits your lifestyle. Step by step, you will learn how to:

- Think like a winner (Part One)

- Eat like a winner (Part Two)

- Train like a winner (Part Three)

- Get back on track, when things get off track, like a winner (Part Four) and, as a result, become a weight loss winner!

The advice, eating and training plans throughout this book have been modelled on the same programs I have provided to thousands of people successful at achieving their weight loss goals. I have included eating plans and an exercise program that you can use to share the same weight loss success that they have.

This book uses calories: 1 calorie is equivalent to 4.2 kilojoules.

Also, buy a couple of exercise books (or one big book) to use as your Food Diary, Activity Diary and Weight Loss Journal—it's important to keep track of your progress and it's great to have to look back! This book also has plenty of space for you to scribble on and use as a workbook.

Ray's three simple steps to shaping up

To achieve weight loss and improve your health instantly, I believe you should follow these three steps:

1. Integrate regular exercise: Set aside time each day for an exercise session as well as increasing the amount of incidental activity you do each day outside of planned exercise, such as housework and taking the stairs over the lift. It doesn't matter how long, even five minutes a day is enough to start improving your health—in fact, I recommend you set yourself a goal of doing a minimum of five minutes every day. This tiny amount is achievable no matter how busy you are. Then, once you've done your five minutes, you can build up to do more. This little mind trick works and I find most people end up doing more. Grab your diary today and schedule in some exercise appointments, even if it's just five minutes.

2. Make subtle diet changes: Don't go to the extremes—making one small change combined with regular exercise will get you losing weight. For example, removing fried foods if you eat out a lot, and cutting down to one glass of wine a night from two glasses, are examples of small changes that will make a huge difference. What small dietary changes could you start with?

3. Get strict: Once Steps 1 and 2 aren't having as big an effect on your weight loss, you then call in the big guns and get tougher with your calorie counting. You may have to reduce your calories, burn more, or both. You can also look at more intense training sessions and personal crackdowns such as eliminating the time spent with negative people. You can learn how to make these changes through the pages of this book and in the eating and training plans found in Parts Two and Three.

PART ONE: THINKING LIKE A WINNER

The first step in this process is to get you thinking like a winner. Before you do this, you need to face the fact that you are overweight, the very real health concerns caused by obesity, understand how you got this way, and why you've failed to lose weight in the past. Then we focus on training your brain to think in a new, positive way and begin to make plans to embark on your weight loss journey.

1. Why care about your weight?

It seems we live in a world obsessed with weight—weight loss TV shows top the ratings, the latest celebrity's weight gain or weight loss take up the covers of magazines on a weekly basis, the news headlines are packed with the latest statistics and research about obesity—there's no escaping the topic! So why is our waistline such a weighty issue? Aside from the fact that the weight loss industry is a multi-million dollar one, it's a big deal in our own personal lives for many reasons: weight is directly linked to our physical, mental and emotional wellbeing. Being overweight or obese puts you at an increased risk of: heart disease, stroke, high blood pressure, type 2 diabetes, some cancers (such as colon and breast cancer), sleep apnoea, gall bladder disease, osteoarthritis and polycystic ovarian syndrome (PCOS).

Common health problems in the obese

Your weight can determine your life expectancy, health and risk of disease. The goal of weight loss is to get you to a healthy weight to give you the best chance possible to live a long, happy and healthy life. Losing weight, even just a small amount, leads to massive improvements in your physical, mental and emotional health:

- Reduces blood pressure
- Lowers LDL (bad cholesterol) cholesterol levels
- Reduces your risk of chronic disease such as heart disease
- Prevents and/or manage type 2 diabetes
- Increases life expectancy
- Improves self-esteem
- Increases energy levels
- Prevent and manage depression and anxiety
- Provides stress relief

Being overweight causes a multitude of health problems:

Insulin Resistance

- Insulin is the main hormone responsible for regulating blood sugar (glucose) levels
- Insulin is secreted from the pancreas in response to elevated blood sugar levels, to remove the glucose from the blood
- Insulin also plays a role in fat storage
- Insulin resistance is where the insulin can't effectively act on the cells to do its job properly, resulting in high sugar levels in the body

Polycystic Ovarian Syndrome (PCOS)

- PCOS is a hormonal condition in women, often accompanied by irregular or absent periods, infertility, acne, excessive hair growth or hair loss, weight gain (especially around the mid section) and difficulty losing weight
- Women with PCOS are more likely to have insulin resistance
- Women with PCOS who are overweight/ obese and inactive are at a greater risk of developing type 2 diabetes

High Blood Pressure (hypertension)

- Blood pressure is the driving force that moves the blood through the circulatory system
- It is expressed as two measurements, such as 120 over 80 (120/80)
- Normal blood pressure is less than 120/80
- High blood pressure is when the pressure exerted by the blood as it's pumped through the arteries is high
- High blood pressure (equal to or higher than 140/90) increases the risk of heart attack, stroke and kidney failure

Sleep apnoea

- Sleep apnoea is an interruption of natural breathing patterns while sleeping
- People with this sleeping disorder stop breathing for periods of time during sleep, waking up repeatedly as a consequence, sometimes hundreds of times in one night
- Being overweight increases the risk of sleep apnoea, especially if the weight is carried heavy around the neck area
- Sleep apnoea is also linked to an increased risk of hypertension and cardiovascular disease (CVD)

High cholesterol

- Cholesterol is a fat-related compound naturally produced in the liver, and is involved in many important bodily functions

- The problem with cholesterol occurs when we consume too many animal products such as eggs, meat and cheese, which can increase the level of cholesterol in the body

- Cholesterol is said to be 'good' or 'bad': the good guys, HDL (high density lipoprotein), clean your arteries and have a protective effect in preventing heart disease; the bad guys, LDL (low density lipoprotein), are associated with an increased risk of heart disease

- High levels of LDL are linked to atherosclerosis (build up of plaque on the artery walls)

- Triglycerides also contribute to your total cholesterol score, and are dangerous bad fats and can be higher in people who drink a lot of alcohol and eat cholesterol-rich foods such as cheeses, fried foods and biscuits

- Your doctor can test your cholesterol and tell you if it's within the normal range

- Regular exercise has been shown to increase HDL and decrease LDL

Heart health

Cardiovascular disease (CVD) refers to heart, stroke and blood vessel disease. CVD is the largest single cause of death in Australia, the UK and the US, and heart disease alone kills more Americans than all cancers each year. Physical inactivity and being overweight are major risk factors for heart disease.

Only 5 Percent!

A weight loss of as little as 5 to 10 percent of your current weight reduces the risk of high blood pressure, type 2 diabetes, high cholesterol and osteoarthritis.

Type 2 Diabetes

- Type 2 diabetes is categorised by high blood sugar levels, because the body isn't using insulin properly

- Type 2 diabetes usually arises as a result of lifestyle factors such as being overweight or obese and inactive

- If not managed, glucose levels become too high and become destructive in the body—increasing the risk of heart disease, stroke, circulatory problems (including potential gangrene and amputation), kidney damage, blindness, impotence and other health problems

- Losing weight and doing regular exercise improve the health implications associated with type 2 diabetes, as well as preventing the disease

A growing problem, type 2 diabetes is an unfortunate side effect of being overweight or obese that can have devastating consequences. Annabel Thurlow, director of Action Diabetes, explains further below:

The International Diabetes Federation (IDF) states that there are 382 million people worldwide currently living with diabetes. This number is projected to reach 592 million people living with diabetes by the year 2035. This is an increase of 55 percent!

Type 2 diabetes (T2DM) is increasing in every country. Diabetes is not selective-anyone can develop diabetes if they have one or more of the risk factors.

The risk factors include:

- Age – the greatest number of people with diabetes are between the age of 40-59 years
- Family history of diabetes
- Overweight
- Unhealthy diet
- High blood pressure
- Ethnicity
- Impaired glucose tolerance is a blood glucose level higher than normal, but below the threshold for diagnosing diabetes
- History of gestational diabetes
- Poor nutrition during pregnancyIf you have one or more of these risk factors then you should see your GP and have a formal diagnostic test to confirm whether or not you have T2DM.

T2DM is often referred to as a disorder of lifestyle! The diagnosis of T2DM requires a change to a person's current lifestyle. Change is often 'challenging' – many of the habits people have, they have been performing for all of their lives. Change can be very rewarding and can completely transform a person's life.

Education is vitally important to anyone with diabetes. At diagnosis a person will be referred to a team of healthcare professionals who are qualified to care for a person with diabetes. Diabetes education is ongoing, as new developments in research prove to be beneficial to the management of diabetes.

There is no cure for T2DM, but with lifestyle intervention, a person can successfully manage their diabetes. Successful management of diabetes requires commitment. As a person loses weight their own insulin starts to work more efficiently and the person's blood glucose levels will improve and be closer to the target range. Overall improved glucose levels will mean that a person has less risk of developing complications from diabetes.

Weight loss and increased physical activity have a great many benefits for a person with diabetes: these include:

- Greater control of diabetes levels
- Reduced need for diabetes medication
- Improvement in blood pressure
- Improved cholesterol levels
- Greater mobility
- Greater sense of well being
- Reduced risk of developing complications from diabetes
- More money in the budget due to reduction in medication

Lower limb pain and injury

- Being overweight places enormous strain on the joints of your lower limbs, such as the knees, ankles and feet; just imagine loading an extra 20 kilograms (44 pounds) or more into a backpack and walking around all day and you might appreciate just how much extra pressure these body parts carry.

- Joint pain is strongly associated with body weight.
- Excess weight is a common cause for many lower limb injuries such as shin splints, patella tracking disorder (unstable tracking of the kneecap) and plantar fasciitis (inflammation of the plantar fascia, which causes severe foot and heel pain).
- Being overweight is a risk factor for osteoarthritis, particularly knee osteoarthritis.
- Reducing weight reduces the load your joints have to withstand.

Establishing and Maintaining a Healthy Lifestyle

Margaret J. Morris, professor of pharmacology at the University of New South Wales, Australia, has kindly shared with me her valuable thoughts on establishing and maintaining a healthy lifestyle and the benefits it has on physical and mental health.

Maintaining a healthy lifestyle is critical for cardiovascular, as well as mental, health. We know that high blood pressure is related to the risk of suffering a stroke or having a myocardial infarction. While our blood pressure is partly determined by our genetic makeup, various lifestyle factors can also affect our blood pressure. Having sensible information to guide us in maintaining a healthy lifestyle is a great help, and there are a number of excellent resources available in that regard (e.g., National Heart Foundation).

Establishing a healthy eating pattern is critical, with low fat, high fibre and low salt choices recommended. Reducing alcohol consumption may also have cardiovascular benefits. One of the most important challenges for those trying to improve their lifestyle is to stay motivated.

Obesity is a major contributor to cardiovascular disease risk, and is a major challenge facing our community. However, the relationship between obesity and high blood pressure is unclear, and could reflect hereditary, environmental (lifestyle), and hormonal factors. Of course, improving diet and increasing physical activity are both important weapons in the fight against obesity, and it is important to combine these strategies for the best outcome. Maintaining a healthy weight into advanced age is also important for optimal health.

2. Are you overweight?

Only you can decide what weight or dress size will make you feel self-confident, vital and energetic. But you have to face the fact that excess weight increases your risk for many health problems. While any weight loss will reduce your risk of disease and chronic illness, your overall goal should be to fall in a healthy weight range. To determine whether your weight is healthy or not, let's look at five methods of measurement:

1. **Weight**

2. **Girth measurements**

3. **Waist circumference**

4. **Body fat**

5. **Body Mass Index**

You can keep a record of these in the Testing Diary in the Appendix.

THE SECRET OF GETTING AHEAD IS GETTING STARTED!

Mark Twain

Weight

This is the one everyone hates. Too much emphasis is placed on weight and it isn't an accurate measure of how much excess fat you carry. You can burn 10 kilograms (22 pounds) of fat but the scales only show you as 5 kilograms (11 pounds) lighter. It happens all the time. When you haven't exercised much and you start a regular program, it can be quite easy to put on a bit of muscle, which weighs more than fat (not to mention changes in body fluid levels). The weight of an individual is a measure of heaviness, not a measure of fatness. This makes it a poor measure of health as the scales cannot determine how much of the person's weight comes from muscle, bones, fluid or fat, and what matters is how much fat a person carries. Weight should only ever be used as a general guide, and never used as a primary measure of health or wellbeing. A more accurate representation would be underwater weighing, to get a picture of how much of the total weight is taken up by body fat, lean mass (consists mainly of muscles, bones and vital organs) and water weight. Water weight represents the amount of weight taken up by water in your body. A measure of water in your body can be very helpful in explaining rapid weight loss or gain.

Many rapid weight loss plans prey on victims who are willing to dehydrate their bodies in order to lose weight. With these plans people lose weight rapidly, but the weight often returns just as fast. However, underwater weighing isn't widely accessible, so a common set of bathroom scales is what most people use. Weigh yourself without shoes and socks, and stand on the scales with feet evenly spaced so the weight is evenly distributed over both feet. Don't weigh yourself more than once a week, and always on the same set of scales for consistency. You can measure your progress more accurately by using a measuring tape to take your girth measurements.

Girth measurements

Because your weight can fluctuate so much—caused by factors such as too much sodium, menstruation, and the amount of fluid you're drinking—an easier way to measure changes in body shape is through girth measurements. All you need is a measuring tape (the kind you use for taking measurements for sewing clothes) to measure the distance around your waist, hips, and thighs. The measuring points can be found at these locations:

Belly fat and heart disease

Having a waist circumference greater than 94 centimetres (37 inches) for males or 80 centimetres (31.5 inches) for females increases your risk of coronary heart disease.

Belly Fat

When extra fat is stacked around the mid-section, your heart has to work harder to force the blood around the body.

Waist: This is the smallest place between your hips and your chest.

Stomach: In line with your navel.

Hips: This is the biggest measurement at the pelvis.

Be sure to keep the tape measure firm, and parallel to the floor. You will measure your improvements against your own measurements (not against an ideal score) and re-take them every 2–4 weeks. This way you can see changes in your body shape and compare them against your previous measurements, instead of someone else's notion of an 'ideal' weight. Another way to see changes in these measurements is to regularly try on an old item of clothing—such as a pair of jeans or pants you can't do up anymore, a dress you can't get past your thighs, or a tight fitting shirt that you can't button up. You can gauge reductions in your waist, hips, and thighs according to how much closer you are to fitting into the item of clothing again.

Waist circumference

The size of your waist is an indicator of abdominal fat—a.k.a. potbelly or beer gut—which is an indicator of your risk of health problems, particularly heart disease. A waist circumference above 94 centimetres (37 inches) for men, and 80 centimetres (31.5 inches) for women, is associated with a greater risk of health problems. Higher than 102 centimetres (40 inches) for men, and 88 centimetres (34.6 inches) for women is associated with serious health risks.

Ideal waist circumference: Less than 94 centimetres (37 inches) for men and less than 80 centimetres (31.5 inches) for women. Another measurement used to assess your risk of obesity-related disease is your waist-to-hip ratio. You get this by dividing your waist circumference by your hip measurement. For example, if your waist was 90 centimetres (35.4 inches) and your hip measurement was 100 centimetres (39 inches), your waist-to-hip ratio will be:

$$90 \div 100 = 0.9$$

The closer the score is to 1.00, the greater the tendency towards the 'android' (apple shape) fat distribution, which is associated with a higher risk of disease. The lower the figure, the greater the tendency towards the 'gynoid' (pear shape) fat distribution and the lower the risk of disease.

Ideal waist-to-hip ratio: Less than 0.9 for men and less than 0.8 for women.

BMI Risk

A BMI value of 23 has been shown to provide the lowest risk of cardiovascular disease, with each digit increase above this point increasing cardiovascular disease mortality by 2 percent.

Childhood Obesity

Research has shown that increased levels of obesity are associated firstly with childhood overweight and obesity but also that those people who gain a large amount of weight between the ages of 18–25 are most at risk for lifetime obesity and the development of medical problems associated with obesity. This is why the rising weights and waistlines of our younger generations causes such a stir in medical circles, as we are seeing an increasing proportion of the population who are at risk of developing disease.

Body fat

The measurement of body fat consists of total fat throughout the body. The most common measures of body fat are taken through skin fold callipers (where someone pinches your skin to separate fat from muscle) and body fat scales. These scales use a method called Bio-electrical Impedance Analysis (BIA) where you stand on a pair of scales and a safe electrical current passes through your body, then—based on this reading, your weight, height, gender and training level—it comes up with a percentage. Leave room for error when using these methods. The distribution of body fat also needs to be looked at: fat stored around the abdomen is dangerous fat. It is associated with a greater risk of disease, in particular heart disease; whereas the fat that women tend to hold around the hips and thighs is far less harmful.

Ideal body fat range: 12 percent for men and 17 percent for women.

	Men	Women
Lean	<12 percent	<17 percent
Acceptable	12–20.9 percent	17–27.9 percent
Mod. Overweight	21–25.9 percent	28–32.9 percent
Overweight	>26 percent	>33 percent

Body Mass Index (BMI)

Body Mass Index is used as a general indicator of obesity. It is used to define overweight, obese and underweight levels. To work out your BMI, divide your weight in kilograms by your height in metres squared.

For example, if you weigh 100 kilograms (220 pounds) and are 185 centimetres (6 foot) tall, the equation would be:

$100 \div (1.85 \times 1.85) = 29.2$ (Overweight)

See *www.raykellyfitness.com* for a calculator.

Ideal BMI: 20–25

	BMI	Obesity Class
Underweight	<18.5	
Normal	18.5 – 24.9	
Overweight	25 – 29.9	
Obesity	30.0 – 34.9	I
	35.0 – 39.9	II
Extreme Obesity	40.0 +	III

Having a BMI above 30 (obese) significantly increases the risk of a wide range of diseases, including heart disease, diabetes, stroke, osteoarthritis, and gall bladder disease. Having a BMI of 26–30 means that your body fat level is greater than recommended (overweight), but your build should be taken into account (i.e. if you carry a large amount of muscle mass you will score an inaccurately high reading).

3. Why are you overweight?

There's often not one simple answer to why someone is overweight, or why your friend can eat chips and chocolate every day and you just have a whiff of these foods and your stomach expands! There's an intricate and complex interplay of elements involved in fat loss, and researchers are finding new reasons every day. Some causes of weight gain that we can bet on:

Lack of incidental activity: Incidental activity is the work you do throughout the day that would not be described as exercise—housework, mowing the lawn, and walking around the house or office, are all examples of incidental activity. It's important to include more incidental activity in your life, as it will help you to burn more calories. Like your exercise sessions, it doesn't have to be hard, just regular. And there's a big pay off to bumping up your movement quota: moving more can increase the calories you burn each day by up to 70 percent, and that's without having to don a pair of sneakers to do a 'workout'!

Less exercise: Because we move less, there's a need to do extra exercise sessions. A hundred years ago, daily chores and living was a lot more manual so there was no need to do an extra 'workout'. Sadly, regular exercise is not common; according to the World Health Organisation (WHO) at least 60 percent of the global population fails to achieve the minimum recommendation of 30 minutes of moderate intensity physical activity daily.

Poor diet: With access to so many unnatural, processed and takeaway foods, it's too easy to make poor diet choices over preparing fresh, wholesome, homemade foods. Thanks to hidden fats, sugars, artificial preservatives and additives, we're consuming too many calories.

Lack of time: We live in such a fast-paced world—career ladders to climb, family commitments to juggle, material standards to live up to—finding the time to exercise and eat healthy, and put ourselves first often takes a backseat.

Poor sleep: Several studies have confirmed that sleep deprivation can cause weight gain. Lack of sleep affects the hormones that are linked to increased appetite and slower fullness signals to the brain.

> ALL THAT WE ARE IS THE RESULT OF ALL THAT WE HAVE THOUGHT.
>
> **Buddha**

Ray's top 10 tips for weight loss

1. Eat a variety of fresh foods, keeping saturated fats, trans fats, sugar and sodium levels low.

2. Exercise each day—even if it's just for five minutes, it all adds up. When exercising, keep your heart rate over 120 beats per minute.

3. Drink more water.

4. Get support. Find someone that you can speak with on a regular basis that understands what you're going through.

5. Be honest: with yourself, with the people who support you, and with your trainer (if you have one).

6. Remove all temptations from your house. You know you'll succumb when you're weak so why have them?

7. Surround yourself with positive people and you too will have a positive outlook.

8. Planning brings success. The goal setting and crisis strategies (as in your contract) help with this.

9. There's no such thing as failure, as long as you've learnt something, so no matter what happens keep moving forward.

10. Respect your own opinion over others. Just because someone else says something it doesn't make it true. You know what you need to do, so just do it.

One study found that those who slept for less than four hours are 73 percent more likely to be obese. Seven to nine hours sleep seems to be the best prescription for weight control.

Medical factors: There can be medical reasons behind a person's weight gain and/or inability to lose weight. Some of these are: underactive thyroid, side effects of certain medications, insulin resistance, Syndrome X, and PCOS. The good news is lifestyle plays a far greater role than medical problems.

Genetics: Genes do influence a person's body type and shape, and scientists are continuing to find more genetic links to obesity. 'Everyone in my family is fat' and 'I can't lose weight because it's genetic' are often overused explanations. But, it's more likely that the diet and lifestyle is inherited from the family rather than some fat gene!

Emotional factors: There are many emotional and mental factors that can cause a person to binge eat and not take care of themselves, such as low self-esteem. Do any of the above reasons for being overweight resonate with you?

How stress makes you fat

Not only does stress compromise your health, it can also cause you to gain weight, and make it hard to lose weight. Stress can sabotage your weight loss efforts in many ways: People who are 'stressed-out' rarely follow a healthy lifestyle such as regular exercise, eating properly, or getting enough sleep. In a bid to deal with stress some people smoke cigarettes, drink alcohol, take other drugs or overwork—all are destructive to our health and weight. Stress is a major cause of binge and comfort eating and is linked to obesity, weight gain and abdominal fat. Studies have identified a link between high cortisol

Stress busters

This week make a point of changing the way you react to stressful situations. Replace negative reactions with positive ones—such as going for a walk or calling a friend to vent your stress. Instead of reaching
for chocolate, grab your Weight Loss Journal. List every activator that you come across in the week. How did you react? Is that how you'd usually react? How could you have reacted better?

(hormone we release in response to stress) levels and the storage of fat around the mid-section. When we encounter a challenging situation our nervous, endocrine (hormone), and immune systems get together to battle the problem. Illness arises when these systems are continually activated. Our immunity levels soon become low and we then become more susceptible to illness and low energy levels, which impacts our ability to be healthy and active.

What is stress?

The phrase 'I'm so stressed' seems to have become part of our everyday vocabulary; but what does stress really mean? When we react strongly to a stressor our bodies produce a number of physiological responses—this is called the 'fight or flight' response. Basically, it's an in-built program designed to get you ready to attack or flee a stressful situation. This sets off a series of responses in the body, for example:

- Heart rate, breathing rate and blood pressure increases
- Blood flow to the organs of the abdomen (such as stomach and intestines) is reduced because digestion is no longer a priority
- Blood flow to skeletal muscles (those needed for 'fight or flight') is increased
- Stored glycogen (blood sugar) is released for quick-releasing energy
- Stored triglycerides (fats) are released to further meet the increased energy demands
- Hormones are secreted—primarily epinephrine (adrenaline) and cortisol.

All of these responses are imperative to 'fight or flight' a genuinely stressful situation, such as fighting off an attacker or running from a burning building, but setting this mechanism off repeatedly in response to everyday stresses, such as meeting deadlines or sitting in traffic, is unnecessary and harmful. Prolonged exposure to stress can lead to physiological symptoms such as insomnia, headaches, gastro-intestinal upset, muscular tension and obesity.

The three components of stress

1. Stress activators

Activators are the situations in life that have the potential to cause us stress. It may be the death of a loved one, an argument with someone, an injury, or just getting caught in traffic.

2. Reactions to activators

Your reaction to the activator has very little to do with the actual situation. It has more to do with your personality and emotional make-up. We each interpret the world and events differently. Our perception is based on our life experience, beliefs, values, and attitude. This means that a situation that one person finds stressful will not be stressful to another. This is because the person experiencing the stress interprets the situation as important to them.

3. Consequences of our reactions

The stress response sets off undesirable physiological changes.

Dealing with stress

When it comes to losing weight, attitude is everything, and attitude is determined by how you think—positive or negative. If your attitude is bad, then you're not likely to eat well or exercise regularly. On the other hand, if you can maintain a good attitude you'll have the strength to overcome any hurdles that get in your way. The way you think determines how you deal with stress. Confronting and resolving stresses is essential for successful weight loss—as well as a happy and healthy life! Each day brings its own challenges, some we breeze through and others test us. When confronted with these challenges we may feel angry, sad, excited, depressed, afraid or anxious. Unless these issues are dealt with, one problem can ruin your week, month, or even years.

You may not be able to control a stressful event from occurring but you can control your reaction to it. Our reactions will define where life will lead us. If you continually see yourself as the victim, then that's exactly what you'll be. But by changing your reaction to the event you reduce the response from your nervous system and the amount of hormones released. We can then get past the initial stress of the event much faster and get on with the job of improving the situation—not to mention save ourselves from the damaging health effects of stress.

Put stress into perspective

Grab your Weight Loss Journal and let's get on top of your stresses. Think of what causes you stress and work through the following questions and points.

1. Is it something from the past? Then it can't be changed, so move on.

2. Is it currently happening? Then what can you do right now to improve the situation?

3. Is it because it could happen in the future? Then it hasn't even happened yet!

4. What is the worst case scenario? What is the likelihood it'll happen?

5. What is the best case scenario? What can you do to improve your chances of a positive outcome?

6. Have a good look at the situation. Is it something that you know will mean very little to you in a month? Does it really deserve the importance you give it?

7. Do you deserve the pain it will cause if you don't do something about it immediately?

Don't self-medicate to soothe stress

All forms of self-medication need to be thrown out. If you have a problem I don't want you to drink, smoke, or eat your way through it. It won't fix the problem; it'll only put off dealing with it. Continuing to self-medicate will also reduce your ability to deal with problems in the future. Overcoming problems is a learned skill. So instead of self-medicating, I want you to replace it with a positive activity like exercise. At least then you'll be gaining something positive (better health) from a negative situation.

4. Finding solutions, not excuses

Chances are you've previously tried to lose weight. In order to be successful this time you need to identify the reasons why it just hasn't worked out before. How many times have you tried to lose weight only to put it back on in half the time it took you to lose it? Do you feel somewhat hopeless when it comes to the thought of losing weight, like you're never going to achieve your weight loss goals? Does the thought of failing stop you from even trying? If you answered yes to any of these questions then you must read on. This is the first step towards changing the way you think—think success, not failure. Replace every excuse you can think of to avoid losing weight with a solution!

Are you afraid to fail?

What if I can't do it? What if I give up after only a few days? What if everyone thinks I'm weak? What if I lose weight and I'm still not happy? What if … what if … what if? Being too scared to fail can make you too scared to try. If you don't feel good about yourself, adding another 'failure' to the equation can reinforce your low sense of self-worth and further cement your 'I'm a failure' belief. The reality of this can be so painful that you want to avoid it. If you do think this way, you're going to have to break through your fear and give it a go. You need to replace your negative 'what ifs?' with positive 'what ifs?' Try this little exercise. Grab your Weight Loss Journal, and write down all of the negative 'what ifs?' and replace them with a positive 'what if?'

- What if I don't succeed? … What would my life be like if I do?

- What if I can't do it? … What if I can?

- What if I lose weight and I'm still not happy? … What if it does make me happy?

- What if … keep going …

Note your feelings when you write the positive 'what if?' Does it fill you with a glimpse of excitement or possibility? Or does it provoke a sense of anxiety? If it's the latter, you may actually be afraid of succeeding.

> CREATE A LIST OF REASONS YOU WANT TO BE HEALTHY AND READ IT REGULARLY!
>
> **Ray Kelly**

Self-sabotage

It sounds like a silly question, but do you really deserve success? Most of you will answer with a firm 'Yes', but do you really believe it? Everyone wants success, but few know how to handle it. It's easy to get comfortable being the person you are, and change could just rock the boat. Self-sabotage is a common occurrence when people lose weight. Often people have a pay-off from being overweight—such as being in a comfort zone or having an excuse to fall back on to explain why things don't go right in their life—so people often sabotage their success without really knowing why; it may seem strange that someone would try to ruin something that they want, but our reasons for staying stuck in a certain situation (or body) can be very powerful.

If you regularly relapse after losing weight, you may be self-sabotaging, and you may need to speak to someone to get to the bottom of your unconscious beliefs. Keeping a journal of your thoughts, feelings and beliefs can also be an easy way to learn more about what makes you tick, if you don't feel comfortable talking to a close person or professional.

Remember, failures aren't a bad thing. You can see them as a positive event because of the lessons they contain. If you have failed to lose weight, now is the time to reflect on why. With each failure, comes a new lesson, and through a series of 'failures' you can keep taking steps to move closer to success.

Finding new ways of thinking

What reasons (sometimes excuses!) have you used in the past, or still use today? This list comes from the patients in my clinics. Write your reasons in your Weight Loss Journal, or tick which of the following reasons apply to you:

- ☐ **Lack of motivation**
- ☐ **Lack of time**
- ☐ **Too expensive**
- ☐ **Sore back/hip/knee/ankle**
- ☐ **Finding clothes to exercise in**

5. Training your brain

Most of us focus our energies on the external when we think of shaping up. We think we have to lift weights to tone up, start a running program to shed pounds, diet to lose weight. It's all about working with the body. Yet how many of us put equal emphasis on working with our minds. You need to train your brain as much as you do your body in order to come up with the winning weight loss strategy. Before we embark on our mental shape-up plan, let's review what we've covered in the previous chapters (write your answers in your Weight Loss Journal).

1. What is my current weight/what are my current measurements?

2. How did I become overweight?

We all have different reasons for becoming overweight. Write down how you've come to be the weight you are today.

3. Why is losing weight and becoming healthier important to me?

You can't expect to be successful unless being healthy is important to you. Why do you really want to lose weight and be healthier?

4. How will it change my life?

There are many positive changes that occur when you lose weight. List the positive changes you expect to happen. Please don't write something like 'I will feel better about myself'. This exercise will work much better if you think of specific situations. For example, what will it be like when you go out? How will you feel when you go shopping? For guys, how will it feel when you take your shirt off at the beach? Don't be afraid to get excited. Be passionate!

Now let's move on to think about what has prevented you from losing the weight you desire to.

Justifying thoughts

The toughest part of being a trainer is trying to decipher some client's version of the truth. I can't tell you how important it is to be honest with your trainer (and yourself). There are people who can help you, but if you're not honest then it just makes it harder to help you reach your goals. I wish I had a dollar for every time I've heard 'I eat healthy, I exercise, but I just can't lose weight'. It seems we can justify just about anything if we want to! The fact is if I had you away from all temptations, and stood with you while you ate and exercised each day then you would lose weight. So let's be blunt: you're just not being honest with yourself. If you're really going to get serious about your weight, you can't fill your mind with justifying lies. You've got to be real. You've got to be honest. You've got to be straight up. Grab your Weight Loss Journal and write down what things you tell yourself to justify your non-committal behaviour. Some common justifying thoughts to get you started (tick any off that apply to you):

- ☐ **One block of chocolate won't hurt**

- ☐ **A hamburger has salad in it so it mustn't be too bad**

- ☐ **We'll have to have take-away tonight because I'm too tired to cook**

- ☐ **I'm just not an exercise person**

- ☐ **I have to have a gym membership to be motivated to workout**

- ☐ **I need a personal trainer to push me**

- ☐ **I don't have the time**

- ☐ **Eating healthy costs too much**

- ☐ **I need snacks in the house because the kids like them**

- ☐ **One night out drinking per week isn't too bad**

- ☐ **My partner brings junk food into the house**

☐ I can't exercise because I have kids

☐ It's too hot/cold outside

☐ I need a sugar hit

☐ I need someone to train with

☐ I'll skip dinner on days I pig out

☐ I'll skip breakfast so I can eat whatever I want later

☐ I have a slow metabolism, so there's no point

☐ If I exercise I can eat whatever I want

☐ I have a sore ankle/knee/elbow/back, etc

☐ I'll exercise tomorrow (yeah, right!)

☐ I have to keep biscuits in the house for when guests pop in

☐ I don't want my kids to miss out on treats so I have to have them in the cupboard

Clean your mental hard drive

Is your brain conditioned the right way to succeed? What kind of thoughts do you keep about your weight loss? Are they positive and self-affirming or negative and self-defeating? Thoughts pop into your head a thousand times a day. They're like daydreams; there's no sense behind them, they just pop in. So should you let them rule your life? Of course not!

Most of us have programmed our brains to think a certain way, and if our mental hard drive isn't full of positive thoughts you'll find it tough to lose weight and maintain it.

DISCIPLINE IS CHOOSING BETWEEN WHAT YOU WANT NOW AND WHAT YOU WANT MOST!

To make sure your thoughts are geared towards success we need to clean this mental hard drive by wiping any of those doubting and negative voices that creep in and try to sabotage your weight loss success. You may not be able to do anything about the negative thoughts popping in, but you can do something about them hanging around. Don't give them any time to settle, just get that thought out of there as soon as it comes in. Then replace it with something you know is true and positive. For example:

Negative self-talk: I'm too tired to go for a walk.

Positive self-talk: I am tired now but I know that when I get back I'll feel much better.

Negative self-talk: It's all too hard.

Positive self-talk: If I push through this I will be much healthier.

Negative self-talk: I'll do it tomorrow.

Positive self-talk: I need to exercise today to stay on track.

Negative self-talk: I'm too exhausted to cook and I feel like pizza.

Positive self-talk: We'll get take-away tonight but I'll eat something healthy.

Now it's your turn … in your Weight Loss Journal, write down the negative thoughts that pop into your head when it comes to losing weight, getting fit, eating healthy, and achieving your goals. Then replace it with a more positive thought. Keep these new thoughts close by for you to refer back to; like training your body, it takes consistency and hard work to get results, so it will be hard work to keep replacing old negative thoughts with new positive ones, so keep at it, until affirming thoughts just happen automatically.

Visualising your way to weight loss

Visualisation is an important tool in success and overcoming your fear of the unknown. It's a very common tool used by most athletes—they see themselves crossing that finish line and standing on the gold medal dais, long before they get there. Visualisation is a lot like daydreaming but you assume much more control. There are many visualisation tools around that have been developed and explained by experts in the field of psychology. If you're interested in exploring the field of visualisation further you could do some research into the subject, invest in a guided audio visualisation CD or see a professional. But you don't have to be an expert in visualisation techniques; it really can be quite quick, simple and easy. A good time to do it is just before going to sleep, but you can do it throughout the day if you'd like. Just find a quiet place, close your eyes, and think about what it would be like to be thinner. A good way to get into the right, relaxed frame of mind is to close your eyes and take 10 long, slow deep breaths, then start on the following:

- How would you look? What are you wearing? What specific parts of the body can you see changes in? How would you feel? What expression can you see on your face? What is your body language?

- How would you act? Can you see the body gestures that show your confidence and pride?

- How would others treat you? Who is around you? What are they saying? How do they look at you?

This is a very powerful tool and really works wonders. Just doing it for five minutes every day can make unbelievable changes to your motivation and confidence. Don't be too concerned if you feel you can't really see it in your mind too well at the start. That's normal. Just like everything else, it takes practice, and the more you practice the better you get. In fact, you'll get to the stage where you can actually hear the sounds, and even the smells will be clear.

Burn your boat!

If you really are committed to losing weight you have to decide that this is it; that there's no turning back to old habits and beliefs and comfort zones. You have to let go of the old you and stay true to the new you!

There's a story about the ancient Greek warriors unwavering commitment to battle: as they would offload from their boats onto their enemy's shore, the first order given by their commanders was 'Burn the boats!'—symbolising their faith and belief that there's no turning back; that we will not need to surrender or retreat because we will overcome adversity and defeat or we will die trying.

Basically, it's about full commitment right from the start. Nothing half-hearted. Just commit to it and see it through. It's this commitment—a new way of thinking—you need to show for weight loss. What ways could you burn the boat as a sign of full-fledged commitment to your weight loss battle?

It could be:

- Clearing out your pantry
- Telling your friends about your goals and telling them that you want to lose weight and don't need anyone tempting you with foods you can't have
- Keeping your goals around for all to see so those that you live and work with can remind you of your commitment
- Throwing your current (or fat) clothes away
- Paying in advance for a gym membership or personal trainer
- Organising to train with a friend
- Commiting yourself to a group for the next fun run (or you can walk it!)
- Making a deal with a loved one: If you exercise each day, they can't smoke!

List any other ways you can make a no-turning-back-commitment to your weight loss in your Weight Loss Journal.

6. Setting sensible goals

Based on all of the information and thoughts you have gathered from working through the questions in this section it's time to start setting a plan of action by setting some concrete goals.

Goal setting is a simple method for designing a successful plan that suits your individual lifestyle. It works because it is designed by you to combat your own personal weaknesses. Successful goal setting covers three types of goals:

Outcome goals

Process goals

Performance goals

Outcome goals

Your outcome goal is what you wish to achieve. As you are trying to lose weight, it may be how much weight you want to lose by the end of the year, or end of the program. It's important to not only state how much you want to lose, but also a time frame. This makes your goal measurable, which makes it easy to see how you're going along the way! Examples of outcome goals:

Outcome goal 1: To lose 8 kilograms (17.6 pounds) in 12 weeks.

Outcome goal 2: To run continuously for 20 minutes by my birthday.

Outcome goal 3: To lower my cholesterol from 6.8 to 5.0 by Christmas.

Outcome goal 4: To make healthy eating for my family and myself a daily habit over the next three months.

Process goals

Process goals are the most important of all. These goals outline exactly what you need to accomplish each day in order to achieve your outcome goals, kind of like a daily checklist. They should not only target how much you eat or exercise, but also your strategies for overcoming negative self-talk and past failures. So go back to the answers you have provided in the previous chapters, as well as the strategies suggested for the list of 'Past Failures' and design your daily goals. Examples of process goals:

Process goal 1: I will burn __ calories in each exercise session, each day (aim for 400–700).

Process goal 2: I will consume __ calories each day (usually between 1200–1800).

Process goal 3: I will eat at least three meals per day.

Process goal 4: I will stick to my meal plan as set by the dietician, reducing my intake of fat, and reducing my portion sizes.

Process goal 5: I will ensure my meals are planned at the start of each week to ensure quality low-fat foods are available to me each day.

Process goal 6: I will increase my incidental activity each day.

I will do this by:

Never using the remote

Playing with my child for at least 15 minutes each day

Participating in at least 15 minutes of housework each day

Parking at the far end of the car park at work and when shopping

Getting up to make my own tea and coffee when at work

Performance goals

Performance goals relate to your exercise regime. Even though any exercise is better than none at all, there are certain standards that will ensure success. Some examples of performance goals:

Performance goal 1: I will exercise ___ days per week. (Hint: 7 is best!)

Performance goal 2: After I warm-up, I will make sure my heart rate is always above ___ beats per minute (bpm) during each training session. (Unless advised otherwise by your physician, this should be at least 120bpm).

Crisis control

You know that no matter how much successful planning you do each week you're likely to have certain situations that may test your resolve. You can think of these as 'crisis situations'. By identifying them you can design a plan to improve your ability to achieve your goals. For example:

Friday afternoon drinks:
I will limit myself to two schooners of light beer.

Dinner with friends on Saturday:
I will call the restaurant in advance and ask them to email/fax a copy of the menu so I can study my options and not make a decision on an empty stomach.

Son's soccer game where I end up eating meat pies and sausage rolls:
I will prepare sandwiches for my lunch.

Rewards

Rewarding yourself when you achieve your goals (short and long-term) not only makes your journey more enjoyable but it's also an important motivational tool. They can provide incentive to keep going when things get tough. Your rewards need to be non-food rewards (sorry!), such as new clothes, a facial, a night-in with your favourite DVD, and so on.

Just finish the sentence: When I do this I will …

Example 1: When I go for six walks this week I will treat myself to a movie with my friends.

Example 2: When I achieve my weight loss goal of 30 kilograms I will take that trek I have always wanted to do.

You can plan your rewards daily, weekly, monthly or yearly. Just jot them down in your Weight Loss Journal and tick them off as you go.

It's now time to put all of your goals down on paper and make a commitment to seeing them through. Use the personal commitment contract to make your goals definite and get everyone around you onboard. It is very important to have at least one person both at work and at home, to support you.

Seeing is believing

As you move your body, imagine the fat being burned up as you train. Actually go into your body and imagine what it would look like to see the fat burning up and disappearing.

See yourself feeling body confident on the beach.

Imagine a sculptor at work with your body. See them carving and chiselling away the bits you don't want and smoothing the edges to create your very own body masterpiece.

See your slim self dressed up and stepping out to a party, and having people acknowledge how great you look.

Personal commitment contract

I, _____, on _____, state that it is my desire to attain the following outcome goals. I enter into this contract with _____, and _____ to confirm these goals and to ask for their support.

My outcome goals are: _____
_____
_____

My process goals are: _____
_____
_____

My performance goals are (optional): _____
_____
_____

My crisis control strategies are: _____
_____
_____

If I achieve these goals I will not only be rewarded with greater health, but also the following rewards: _____

_____

_____

Signed: Workplace support _____

Signed: Home support _____

Signed: Me _____

Keep your contract somewhere you can revisit each day to
remind you of your commitment.

PART TWO: EATING LIKE A WINNER

Now that you've got your brain geared to thinking like a winner, documented the reasons you've failed to lose weight previously and made a commitment to embark on a weight loss journey; it's time to look at the way you eat. 'Going on a diet' is usually the first thing on our checklist when we put a plan in place to lose weight, but we're going to redefine the meaning of a diet! Diets are probably the most talked-about and misunderstood element of weight loss. With so much information out there in the form of diet books, the media and friends advice, it can be downright confusing to know which diet is best. In this part I show you how weight is lost, what foods are the best type for weight loss, and how to reduce your food intake using the 500-calorie-cutting Plan or my meal plan, with recipes for meals in the plans in Chapter 11.

> A BRISK WALK
> FOR 20 MINUTES
> BEFORE BREAKFAST
> IS A GREAT WAY
> TO FIRE UP YOUR
> METABOLISM.
>
> **Susie Burrell**

7. The weight loss equation

This is a concept that is usually taught to people when they first start their weight loss journey. I have always found it to be a great way to teach people how to control their food intake (portion size as well as total intake), and, more importantly, how to increase the amount of exercise they're doing. Losing weight is all about calories in versus calories out. The weight loss equation states that you need to burn more calories than you eat—this is called making a caloric deficit.

Calories in > calories out, leads to weight gain

Calories in = calories out, leads to weight maintenance

Calories in < calories out, leads to weight loss

But it's not as simple as subtracting the calories you eat from the amount you burn during exercise; there's another factor involved in the energy equation: metabolism.

Metabolism matters

In order to lose weight we need to make sure we have a calorie deficit after each day by consuming fewer calories than we burn. But what exactly is a calorie?

In actual fact, a calorie is a unit of work and energy. One calorie is the amount of heat required to raise the temperature of 1 gram of water by 1°C. Almost all the calories derived from the food we eat are eventually converted to heat, which you can think of as energy. Heat is lost, or energy is produced, during nearly every activity in every cell of the body—when muscles contract, when energy is formed and stored in the body, when energy is broken down as a fuel, and even when your muscles are repairing themselves.

These bodily functions are part of what we refer to as metabolism.

Basal metabolic rate (BMR)

Metabolism is a blanket term for resting metabolism or basal metabolic rate (BMR). The true definition of BMR is: the minimum rate of metabolism for an individual at rest who is not digesting or absorbing food. So your metabolism is the sum of all the chemical reactions that take place in the body to sustain life—breathing, heart rate, cell renewal and so on—separate to any physical activity you do.

Muscle magic

For every half a kilo (one pound) of muscle you gain, your resting metabolic rate can increase by up to 50 calories a day! Over one week, that's a total of an extra 350 calories (equivalent to two schooners of beer or four standard glasses of wine) you've burnt off without lifting a finger!

You can think of your metabolism as your body's fire: the more logs you add, the more you keep it burning. The higher your metabolism, the more calories you burn and the better fat burner you become. Conversely, add too little wood to the fire by eating too few calories (less than 1200 calories) and you drop your metabolic rate and burn less calories—not good for weight loss. The trick is to find the right balance between getting enough fuel to keep up your energy and metabolism, but not too much to sabotage your weight loss and metabolism. You want to keep adding as many logs as you can to your metabolic fire in order to burn more energy and fat over the course of each day. So where do these 'logs' come from? Some examples of metabolic mobilisers:

- High intensity exercise, which raises your metabolic rate post workout

- Resistance training to build muscle tissue, as the more muscle you have the higher your metabolism

- Eating small meals often, which raises your metabolic rate because eating has a thermogenic (creates heat) effect

- Eating some spicy foods, which can create

Ray's 5 cornerstones of weight loss:

Increase activity—walk the dog, take the stairs, clean the house, walk to buy the newspaper and so on

Exercise every day, even if it's just walking

Control your fat and sugar intake

Maintain variety in your exercise and diet

Hang around positive people.

heat and raise your metabolism, such as capsaicin found in chillis—although this has a very small effect.

How do we burn calories?

The three components to the 'calories in versus calories out' equation are: metabolism, exercise, and diet. If you want to lose fat, it usually comes down to the tried and true energy equation. There really is no magical fat burning program, pill, eating plan or gadget. You just need to move more and eat less! It really is that simple. You can do this with three simple rules:

1. **Cutting down food intake:** I'd like to add a little more to this: Cutting down processed food intake!

2. **Increasing physical activity:** Good health and weight management will not be found without regular exercise. This does not necessarily mean you need some form of organised physical activity. You just need to move more, which takes us to the third point.

3. **Decreasing time spent in sedentary activity:** The effect of this is often underestimated. It sounds crazy but many people think that if they exercise for one hour then they can get away with sitting around for the rest of the day. The truth is that you can burn more calories by 'moving more' throughout the day than you can through a structured exercise regime.

So all of this sounds simple right? So why do so many of us find it so hard to lose weight? For some, the process of weight loss isn't always as simple as 'calories in versus calories out' (researchers are

Rate of weight loss

It takes a caloric deficit of approximately 7700 calories to lose 1 kilogram (about 2 pounds) of fat. So theoretically, if you ate 77 less calories every day or burnt 77 extra calories every day, it would take 100 days to lose 1 kilogram; and if you ate 770 less calories a day or burnt the same amount, it would take ten days to lose 1 kilogram. But it doesn't always work out exactly like this: some people lose weight faster than others and some people will lose weight in inconsistent amounts. So don't be put off if you don't see the same amount of weight come off every week.

finding out about new causes of obesity all the time such as genetic and hormonal factors), but for most of us it is as simple as eating less and moving more.

I'm not suggesting you become a slave to a calculator and calorie-counting book, rather recommending it as a good place to start to gauge your food intake and the amount of exercise you're doing. Most people overestimate the amount of activity and exercise they do and underestimate the amount of calories they consume. Now it's time to get truthful about how many calories you eat and burn.

How many calories are you burning during physical activity?

You can measure calories burned during exercise and general activity by calculating METs (short for Metabolic Equivalent). We can use METs to calculate how much oxygen we consume completing an activity. A MET is a measure of the amount of energy required to perform an activity. Because we know that 1 MET is equivalent to 1.2 calories per minute, we can work out the amount of calories an activity burns. The formula below takes into account bodyweight (remember, calories burnt through exercise vary according to factors such as body weight). To work out how many calories you're burning doing an activity:

0.0175 x METs x bodyweight x time (minutes)

So if a 100-kilogram man took a brisk walk (4 METs) for 30 minutes, he is burning the following:

0.0175 x 4 x 100 x 30 = 210 calories

Common activities and their MET value:

Running (9.5 km/hr)	10
Walking (5.5 km/hr)	3.8
Cycling (20 km/hr)	8
Swimming (freestyle, slow/moderate pace)	7
Raking the lawn	4.3
Scrubbing floors	3.8
Ironing	2.3

Weight loss FAQ

Q: What about diet shakes?

A: Unless you have restricted mobility due to illness or injury and can't exercise, they are not a good long term option. It teaches you nothing about lifestyle change so the weight will often come back once you go off the shakes. They can be used as a snack, or as a kick start for rapid weight loss. Make sure you choose one that's nutritionally balanced and comes with an eating plan, exercise program and ongoing education and support.

Q: What about diet pills?

A: Definitely not! They provide no education on lifestyle change so the chances of long term success is quite low. Some side effects are also quite serious, such as nausea, wakefulness, diarrhoea, increased heart rate and blood pressure, and dizziness.

Weight training (high intensity)	6
Circuit training	8
Boxing (bag)	6

To get the MET value of other activities, see http://prevention.sph.sc.edu/tools/docs/documents_compendium.pdf. You can also use an automatic calculator on www.raykellyfitness.com. Type in your weight, exercise intensity and type of workout and it does the calculating for you.

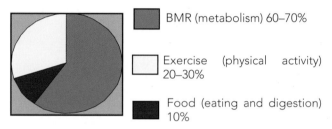

- BMR (metabolism) 60–70%
- Exercise (physical activity) 20–30%
- Food (eating and digestion) 10%

Total Metabolic Rate (TMR)

Your TMR (also commonly referred to as your TDEE or Total Daily Energy Expenditure) is the total amount of calories you require to fuel all daily activities. So we've looked at metabolism and its contribution to your TMR, but what about the other factors that make up your TMR?

This breakdown shows you two important factors: physical activity is the part of your TMR you have most control over and your BMR (Basal Metabolic Rate) is the largest contributor to your TMR.

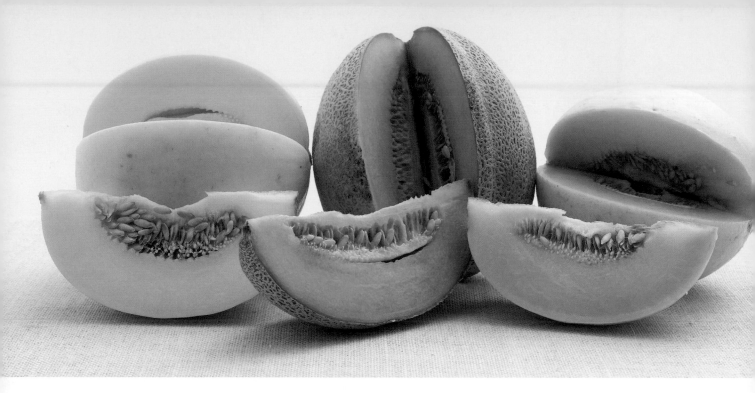

So if physical activity is the largest influence to our TMR that we have control over, you can see why exercise and activity is so important! And not only does it bump up the calories you burn, it also increases your BMR, so you can see why exercise and activity are doubly important!

How many calories are you burning each day?

You can use a calculator to get your BMR and TMR on my site, *www.raykellyfitness.com*. Or you can work it out on your own using the following Mifflin calculation.

Step 1: Calculate your basal metabolic rate (BMR)
Men: (10 x weight in kg) + (6.25 x height in cm) – (5 x age) + 5 = BMR in calories
Women: (10 x weight in kg) + (6.25 x height in cm) – (5 x age) – 161 = BMR in calories
For example, if we want to find the BMR of a 30-year-old, 70-kilogram woman who is 160cm tall:
(10 x 70) + (6.25 x 160) – (5 x 30) – 161 = 1389 calories
The woman's BMR is 1389. So this means she needs 1389 calories to sustain her metabolism, basically

everything she does to live, breathe and function, outside of physical activity.
The next step is to find out how many extra calories she needs to sustain the extra physical activity she does.

Step 2: Calculate your Total Metabolic Rate (TMR)
Of course, we burn more calories than just our BMR. How many more depends on how active you are:

- If you lead a sedentary lifestyle (little or no exercise, desk job) = BMR x 1.2

- If you are only lightly active (light exercise/sports 1–3 days/week) = BMR x 1.375

- If you are moderately active (moderate exercise/sports 3–5 days/week) = BMR x 1.55

- If you are very active (hard exercise/sports 6–7 days/week) = BMR x 1.725

- If you are extremely active (hard daily exercise/sports and physical job or 2 training sessions a day) = BMR x 1.9

So continuing on with our example for our 70-kilogram woman, if she has a sedentary lifestyle, the calculation would be.
BMR x 1.2
1389 x 1.2 = 1666.8

So her TMR (the amount of calories she needs to sustain everything her body does in a day) is 1667 calories. If she wanted to lose weight, she would need to make a calorie deficit by eating less than 1667 calories a day. If she was to be lightly active, she would multiply her BMI x 1.375, which would make her TMR 1910 calories. But a more accurate way is to use the sedentary calculation and then add the calories you burn from any extra exercise or activity you do.

So if our 70-kilogram woman decided to take up some exercise and do a 30-minute brisk walk (burns approximately 147 calories) every day, she would add this amount to the sedentary calculation: 1667 + 147 = 1814 calories. This means she now burns 1814 calories each day, and would need to eat less than this amount in order to lose weight.

Let's look at how to measure the number of calories burned through physical activity.

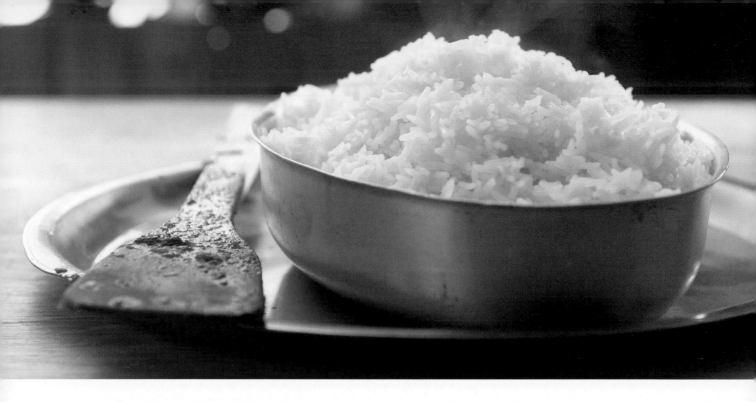

8. Understanding food

Okay, we've talked a lot about calories out (calories burned through metabolism, activity and exercise). Now it's time to talk about calories in (calories consumed through food).

Foods consist of three main nutrients (macronutrients): carbohydrates, proteins and fats:

- Fats are the most energy dense with 9 calories coming from 1 gram

- Protein and carbohydrates both provide 4 calories per 1 gram

- Alcohol yields 7 calories per 1 gram, but these are 'empty calories' meaning they have no nutritional value.

Knowing this information gives you a quick way of measuring the total calories provided from any group. For example, when you're reading the nutritional label on a bottle of full-fat milk and you see that it contains 4g of fat per 100ml, that doesn't sound too unhealthy until you do the calculations:

4g x 9 = 36 calories. There are 66 calories in 100ml of milk and 36 of those calories come from fat, so that means that 53 percent of your calories will come from fat!

Let's look at the three macronutrients in more detail.

Carbohydrates

If you've ever been on a diet, you've surely heard all about carbs (short for carbohydrates). Cutting carbs became so popular in recent years—think Atkins, The Carbohydrate Addict's program, South Beach, the 'no carbs after 2pm' rule—as the certain way to shed pounds. This has made many people afraid of carbohydrates—you could say we have become a generation of carbo-phobics! Well, we need to reverse our way of thinking, because carbs are not the enemy. It's when you have too many carbs that they become the enemy,

Why do I need carbohydrates?

Although the body gets energy from all three macronutrients—carbohydrates, protein and fat— carbohydrates are the body's preferred source of energy. And what needs to be remembered is that not all carbohydrates are created equally. To begin with, a carbohydrate is any food source that, when broken down into a simpler and more useful form by the body, is converted into glucose (blood sugar). Because carbohydrates are the body's main source of energy, we need a steady supply throughout the day. The problem is that as our weight increases it can become increasingly more difficult to process carbs. This makes it very important that we reduce the amount of carbs we eat as well as choose the right ones. Most chemical reactions within the body require glucose. For those looking to make healthier choices for their bodies, it is paramount to understand the differences between simple and complex carbohydrates, processed and unprocessed carbohydrates, and refined and whole carbohydrates, along with the best food sources of each.

YOU CAN'T OUT-EXERCISE A BAD DIET

Carbohydrates are an important source of fibre (which is simply indigestible carbohydrate chains), which is essential for good health and reducing the risk of some cancers such as colon cancer, heart disease, diabetes, and gastrointestinal disorders.

these foods; instead, by consuming them in conjunction with a low GI food or in small portions you lower the overall ranking.

The glycaemic load (GL) can be a better measure than GI as it ranks the GI based on a typical portion size rather than the 50 grams of carbohydrate used to test the GI of foods, so even though a high GI food such as a carrot rank high on the scale, 50 grams of carbohydrates equates to about 1 kilogram of carrots—you're not likely to eat this amount at once unless you're Bugs Bunny—so if eaten in a small portion the overall effect on blood glucose levels is not so great. This means a food with a high GI but a low GL such as carrots is still a good choice.

- Foods with a GL of 20 or over are high GL

- Foods with a GL between 11 and 19 are moderate GL

- Foods with a GL of 10 or less are low GL

To keep things simple, here are some ways to lower the GI of a food: add a little olive oil, add some legumes, add low-fat cheese or yoghurt, add more fibre or stick to just a half a cup of the food.

How much carbohydrate should I have in my diet?

I suggest you have around 40 percent of your daily calorie intake from healthy carbohydrate sources. Unhealthy simple carbohydrate choices include soft drinks, cakes, cookies, donuts,

Best carbs

Vegetables, Nuts, legumes, beans & seeds

Wholegrains

Fruits and some fruit juices

Is bread bad?

Bread is the first thing that usually comes to mind when weighing up the pros and cons of eating carbohydrates to lose weight. Bread isn't bad in itself. As with complex and simple carbohydrates, it's about how much and what type of bread you eat. When trying to lose weight it is best to remove breads initially, but if you must, choose breads that are as close to their natural state as possible, which means they have no artificial ingredients or sugar added to them. A simple rule: buy the heaviest bread you can find. If it's light, white and fluffy stay away—this equals nasty, processed, bleached and all the goodness gone. If it's dark, heavy and grainy and sliced thin then it's most likely okay.

chocolate, and candy. These food items can be found almost everywhere and it's okay to have a little bit now and then; the problems arise from eating these processed and refined simple carbohydrates on a regular basis.

How carbohydrates can help you lose weight

Carbohydrates can assist weight loss in the following ways:

- They're essential for maintaining stable energy levels throughout the day—this is a must if you're going to be energetic enough to make activity and exercise a part of your everyday life

- You need to eat less energy than you burn in order to lose weight, and it's harder to consume too many calories from high fibre carbohydrate sources as opposed to a diet high in fat

- Complex carbohydrates keep you fuller for longer

- Low GI carbs are digested more slowly so you're not ravenous, searching for more carbs, soon after

- Low GI meals have less chance of causing an oversupply of glucose and insulin, which means less chance of turning excess glucose into fat and depositing it in the fat cells

- Fibre-full carbohydrates help keep blood sugar levels steady to prevent cravings.

Best carbohydrate choices for weight loss

Whenever you sit down for a meal try to ensure that your plate has at least one of these natural-state carbohydrates on it:

Vegetables: Choose leafy green vegetables most of the time, and rotate your coloured vegetables each week to ensure variety. An easy rule is to choose at least one vegetable from every colour of the rainbow each week.

Nuts, legumes, beans and seeds: Are all excellent choices when opting for unprocessed complex wholegrain carbohydrates.

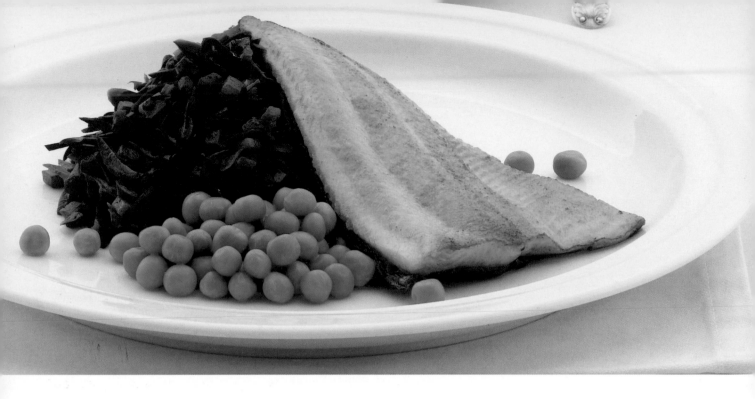

Wholegrains: Examples include 100 percent wholewheat flour products, unprocessed oats, millet, and brown rice. Most of the time, choose brown colours over white colours, which have been refined—such as wholemeal pasta over white pasta. And look for foods that have grains left in, such as 9-grain bread/crackers over white bread/crackers.

Fruits and some fruit juices: These are healthy simple carbohydrate choices. Whole fruits contain an added punch of high fibre, especially when consumed with the skin. Whereas fruit juices are good sources of nutrients but should only be consumed in small quantities and should always come from a 100 percent fruit juice source—it's too easy to consume too many calories from fruit juice, as one glass of orange juice contains 100–120 calories, as opposed to one orange which contains 70 calories.

Protein

Protein can be found in virtually all regions of the body including the muscle, bone, blood, hormones, antibodies and enzymes. Its uses within the body are wide reaching.

Best protein

Grains	Fish
Legumes	Lean meats
Nuts/Seeds	Eggs
Fruit and vegetables	Low-fat dairy
Soy products	

Why do I need protein?

Protein is seen as the body's building blocks—it builds and repairs all body tissues such as skin and muscles, is a major component of enzymes and hormones and is needed for wound repair, balancing fluids and a healthy immune system.

Complete and incomplete proteins

As with the other macronutrients (fat and carbohydrates) there are good protein sources and 'just-okay' protein sources. Let's take a look at the differences. For starters, protein is made of amino acids linked together. There are approximately 20 amino acids that the body requires—some of them the human body can manufacture itself while other amino acids the body must receive from food sources. The latter are known as essential amino acids—essential because it's essential that you include them in your diet. Most animal proteins (meat, fish, poultry, eggs and dairy) are considered 'complete proteins'. It's important that the body receives a full complement of these 20 amino acids in order to function properly. For this reason, eating protein from a wide variety of sources is critical.

Incomplete proteins are those that come from plant sources such as nuts, seeds, wholegrains, legumes and vegetables and most do not contain all of the essential amino acids. For this reason they are labelled 'incomplete proteins'. However, by properly combining several incomplete proteins you can adequately supply the body with all of the amino acids—even the essential ones—without eating protein from animal sources; for example, eating rice with beans or peanut butter on wholegrain bread. This allows vegetarians to still get all the protein they need without breaking their eating habits.

How much protein should I have in my diet?

Adequate and quality protein in your daily diet can dramatically increase the quality of your health. Depending on your activity levels and speed of your metabolism, you may need more or less protein than someone of the same body type and size. I recommend that your daily diet consist of approximately 40 percent protein.

The Recommended Daily Intake (RDI) for protein is 0.8–1 grams of protein for every 1 kilogram (2.2 pounds) of body weight. Additionally, if you are pregnant, recovering from an illness or participate in high levels of physical activity your protein requirements may be greater than the above number.

The average adult with moderate activity levels needs approximately 50–65 grams of protein per day. (Keep in mind that your specific needs are based on your weight, your activity level, your overall general health and your metabolism.) If you know how to read food labels you'll be able to follow your daily protein intake simply by keeping track of what you are eating and how many grams of protein you consume with each meal. Additionally, here are some examples of how much protein some common foods contain:

- 250ml (8¾fl oz) of low-fat milk has approximately 11g of protein

- 1 thick slice of reduced-fat cheese has approximately 9g of protein

- 100g (3½oz) of chicken breast has approximately 25g of protein

- 1 cup (200g) cooked beans has approximately 9g of protein

- 1 serving of vegetables has approximately 1–3g of protein.

For most people in Western countries it's not difficult to reach their recommended protein intake daily. In fact, just by eating one serving of meat each day chances are that you have satisfied 50 percent of your protein requirement for that particular day!

How protein helps you lose weight

High protein diets have been the rage in recent years—popular ones are the Atkins and CSIRO diets. There is evidence that

> NEVER SKIP BREAKFAST; IT SETS UP YOUR DIET FOR THE ENTIRE DAY.
>
> **Susie Burrell**

diets high in protein help people to lose weight initially, as opposed to the 'low calorie' approach. However, researchers have found that the amount of weight lost in those on a high protein diet versus a low calorie diet is the same after 12 months. Having adequate amounts of protein helps you lose weight in the following ways:

- Protein has been shown to stave off hunger and reduce cravings

- You burn calories eating protein: it takes almost two times the energy to break down protein than it does carbohydrates

- Studies have shown that a high-protein meal makes you feel full faster.

A warning on high protein diets

Excessive protein intake has been linked to: osteoporosis, as calcium excretion is accelerated with higher intakes of protein, unless adequate calcium is supplemented; and kidney disease, as the kidneys are responsible for excreting the products of protein metabolism in the urine, which places excess strain on the kidneys.

Best protein choices for weight loss

Choose protein sources that have had the least amount of processing done to them as possible. In other words, if you have to make the choice between ice cream (which has been processed and had additional ingredients added to it) and milk, choose a glass of milk, which is closest to its natural form, if your goal is to eat protein from a dairy source.

Eat a wide variety of protein sources on a daily basis to receive the proper spectrum of essential amino acids along with other healthy nutritional components. Some good sources include:

Grains: Barley, oats, brown rice, wholegrain pasta, wholewheat bread, cornmeal.

Legumes: Beans, lentils, peas, soybeans.

Nuts/Seeds: Sunflower seeds, sesame seeds, all nuts—such as walnuts, almonds, pecans, and spreads made from these nuts and seeds.

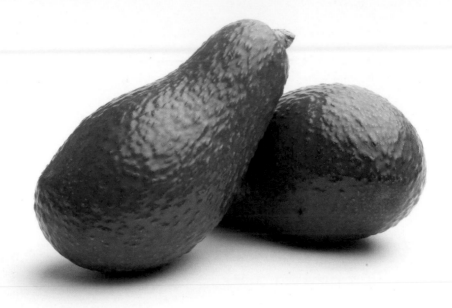

Animal foods: Fish (fresh and tinned), lean meats (beef, pork, poultry), eggs, low-fat dairy (milk, yoghurt, cheese).

Soy products: Tofu and low-fat soy milk.

Note: to assist weight loss and heart health look for lean protein, such as lean meats—the less white fat you see in the meat, the better. Fish is a great source of protein because it doesn't have the high saturated fat of most meats; instead it contains healthy fat.

Fats

The topic of fat in nutrition has been a controversial subject for many years: some say that fat is good so eat all you want while others claim that fat is bad and should be eliminated from the diet completely. During the 1980s and beyond, the low-fat diet was recommended, which instilled fear that eating fat made you fat. This is not entirely true. We need fat in our diets—good fat that is. Bad fats we can do without and too much fat, of any kind, is not healthy for us either.

Why do I need fat?

Fat is a very important macronutrient in human beings; without it we would be unable to absorb, process and utilise the fat soluble vitamins: A, D, E, and K. Additionally, fat is essential for nerve function, for the manufacturing of many hormones, acts as an energy source, cushions our internal organs and insulates us against the external elements. So as you can see fat is certainly necessary in our diet … but what kind?

Good fat versus bad fat

If you watch even a little bit of TV or read magazines you will have surely heard that there are a wide variety of different types of fats—some good, some bad. The good fats are the unsaturated kind: monounsaturated, polyunsaturated and essential fatty acids (omega-6 and omega-3 fatty acids). The bad fats are the saturated fats and trans fatty acids.

To put it succinctly: stay away from bad fats and stick to good fats—in moderation, of course!

Saturated and trans fats

Saturated fats are those that are solid or semi solid at room temperature. They include the fat found in meat, poultry, and dairy products (such as butter). Palm, coconut and palm kernel oils are also considered saturated fats.

Trans fatty acids have come under increased scrutiny lately with many countries calling for a ban on them. Trans fatty acids are unsaturated fats that act in a similar way to saturated fats in the body. Unlike unsaturated fats, trans fats are bad as they have been forced into their unnatural state through a manufacturing process termed 'partial hydrogenation'. The body has a very hard time processing these non-natural fats, so keep them out of your diet completely! Trans fats are commonly found in pre-prepared commercial goods like fries, pastries, pies and biscuits, as well as most margarines. Trans fats are also found naturally, but in small amounts, in some meats, butter and dairy products.

Polyunsaturated, monounsaturated and essential fatty acids

Good fats—monounsaturated, polyunsaturated and essential fatty acids (in particular omega-3) are considered 'heart healthy' fats and should replace other unhealthy fats in your diet whenever it's feasible. Good fats have been shown to lower blood cholesterol and reduce the risk of heart disease.

Polyunsaturated fats are found in vegetable oils such as safflower and sunflower, fish, fish oils, some nuts and seeds and wholegrains, and include omega-3 and omega-6 essential fatty acids (so it's essential you include them in your diet). Omega-3 fats have received lots of attention in recent years for their numerous health benefits— helping alleviate the symptoms of depression, anxiety, arthritis and inflammatory conditions. Great sources include flaxseed, hemp seed, soybeans, walnuts, linseed, dark-green leaves and many forms of cold water fish such as salmon. Monounsaturated fats can be found primarily in avocado, canola, peanut and olive oils and nuts. Margarines and spreads made from unsaturated fats, are usually okay providing they're free of trans fatty acids.

Best fats

Wholegrains

Leafy greens

Olive and canola oils

Oily fish: tuna, salmon, mackerel, sardines, trout, herrings

Flax seeds/flax oil

Nuts and seeds

Unprocessed, all-natural peanut butter

Avocado

Olives

How much fat should I have in my diet?

It's recommended you receive no more than 30 percent of your daily calorie intake in the form of fats, with less than 10 percent coming from saturated fats and consuming a balance between polyunsaturated and monounsaturated fats.

How fats can help you to lose weight

- Omega-3 has been shown to boost metabolism and fat burning capability.

- Fats, like complex carbohydrates and lean protein, keep you satisfied for longer.

- Studies have shown that a dieting group who includes healthy fats, such as olive oil, in their diet, stick to their diets for longer and have better weight loss results than dieters eating a low-fat diet of the same calorie amount.

- Fat increases the satiety factor, helping you to feel satisfied faster.

Best fat choices for weight loss

When making fat choices for health and weight loss, opt for vegetable, grain, fish or seed types of fat.

Limit your intake of fatty meats and poultry as well as high fat dairy products and foods that are cooked or fried in saturated oil. Foods that are processed (and typically not good for you) will usually contain high levels of saturated fats and trans fatty acids. Start reading food labels! Label reading is a tried and true method of recognising which foods are good and bad for you. If the label indicates a high quantity of any bad fat get rid of it and choose an option with heart healthy fats.

Reading food labels

To really get on top of your food choices you will need to become a savvy label reader. The hardest thing about eating healthy is often knowing which product to buy—that's why I say to keep it simple and buy fresh, unpackaged foods. However, there are many healthy products that are packaged, but with so many products on the market that claim to be great for our health, who can you trust? Unless you know how to tell the difference between them they can all look the same. To make the right choices you need to read the nutritional information labels, ingredients list, and decipher marketing claims such as '90 percent fat free'.

Nutritional information table

The nutrition information panel is where you can find all you need to know about what's in the product.

When comparing foods you need to take into consideration sugar, salt (sodium), fat, and fibre. We need to eat more fibre and less sugar, fat, and salt. To make it easier to compare products, always use the 'Per 100g (3 ½oz) 'rather than the 'Per Serving'. This is because the 'Per Serving' varies between manufacturers and products.

The following are large amounts per 100g (3½oz) :

30g of sugars

30g of fat

12g saturated fat

600mg of sodium

The following are small amounts per 100g (3½oz) :

4g of sugars

3g of fat

<1g saturated fat

120mg sodium

Fats are listed as 'total' fat and 'saturated' fat. When trying to lose weight it's best to stick to foods that are low in total and saturated fat.

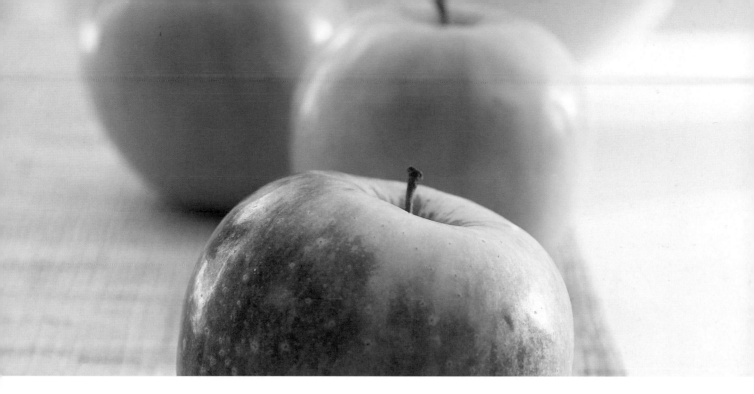

Ingredients list

The ingredients list is a listing of all the ingredients in a product. It lists them from largest quantity to smallest quantity, by weight. Here is an example from a tub of strawberry yoghurt:

Ingredients: Skim milk, Milk, Concentrated skim milk, Sugar, Fruit, Live Acidophilus and Bifidus cultures, Thickener, Gelatine, Flavour, Food Acids (296, 330, 332), Natural colour (120).

So in this example, skim milk is the greatest ingredient by weight. You'll also notice numbers, too, but what do they mean?

Food additives

Ingredients lists must include food additives, which are usually written as numbers. A food additive is any substance that is added to food to preserve or alter the foods taste, appearance, texture or shelf life. Additives may be from nature or be synthetic (artificial). There is a lot unknown about the effects of additives, and many additives have been found to cause adverse reactions such as skin rashes, irritability, headache, and hyperactivity. To learn more about which ones are potentially harmful and which ones are deemed okay, you can buy little pocket books to take with you when you go shopping.

This can be time consuming, but well worth the effort. Once you know what to look out for, shopping becomes a much faster process.

Hidden ingredients

The other things you need to watch out for on the ingredients list are fat, sugars and salts listed under different names, such as:

Fat: Palm oil, vegetable oil, lard, butter, margarine, cream, copha, or animal fat.

Sugar: Raw sugar, brown sugar, cane sugar, sucrose, fructose, lactose, honey, glucose, dextrose, golden syrup, malto-dextrin.

Salt: Sea salt, rock salt, sodium chloride, vegetable salt, and monosodium glutamate (MSG).

Don't be misled by nutritional claims on labels!

Sometimes marketers make certain claims in a bid to make their product sound healthier than it really is. Some common claims:

90% Fat Free! Foods that are 90 percent fat free still contain 10 percent fat and could still contain many calories in the form of sugar.

Light: The term 'light' doesn't necessarily mean that the product is low in fat. They could be referring to the colour, texture or taste.

Low Cholesterol: Although some products are low in cholesterol they can still be high in fat and this is what should be considered if you are trying to lose weight.

Reduced Fat: This doesn't necessarily mean that it's low in fat. The fat content could have been reduced from 90 percent to 60 percent.

Baked Not Fried: Again, this doesn't necessarily mean that it's low in fat. It can mean that the fat was added to the product before baking rather than being fried in the fat.

Sugar Free: This doesn't mean that it's low in carbohydrates and/or fat and can have a high calorie count. It's also likely to contain artificial sweeteners such as aspartame which can exacerbate our hunger, by sending the wrong signal to our minds that we're eating something sweet but there isn't any sugar, so our body starts calling out for the sugar, making us crave it more.

No Added Sugar: May still have a high sugar and calorie content in the form of fruit (fructose).

9. Eating for weight loss

What's the first thing that comes to mind when you want to lose weight and make changes to your body? I need to go on a 'diet'.

If you've been on lots of diets, had success with some but felt frustrated and blameful because you put the weight back on, you need to assess your eating habits.

The word diet usually sends us into panic mode and we feel depressed before we've even started! Take a moment to reflect on what happens to your body when you think of going on a diet. What emotions pop up? What thoughts enter your mind? Here are some of the common thoughts and feelings that surface:

- Deprivation
- Starvation
- Boredom
- Depression
- Frustration
- Anger
- Resistance
- Difficulty

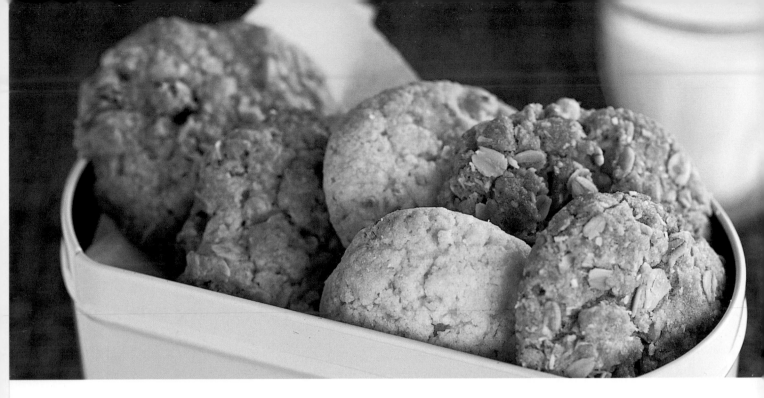

Conversely, so-called 'good' foods can lull us into a false sense of security, leading us to eat as much as we like—guilt free! But when it comes to your weight, the phrase 'You can't have too much of a good thing' couldn't be further from the truth: eat too much 'good' food and you will still gain weight.

Think of 'bad' or 'fattening' foods as 'sometimes' foods, and 'good' foods as 'most-of-the time' foods. And remember, whether it's 'good' or 'bad', eat too much of it without burning it off, and you will gain weight.

Emotional (over)eating

More often than not, finding the successful eating plan for weight loss is more about discovering 'why' you eat, rather than the 'way' you eat. For many, emotional eating is a major roadblock when it comes to sticking to a healthy eating plan. There are many ways we feed our emotions with food, all to make us feel better. We often eat to get comfort when we feel:

- Bored

- Stressed

- Sad

- Anxious

- Depressed

- Lonely

- A lack of love

- Low self-worth

- Unwilling to face our problems.

You can also eat in response to positive emotions, such as eating for enjoyment or as a reward. Until you understand your direct relationship with food and how you use food to deal with things, you can go on any diet with the strongest willpower, but your emotional pattern with food will win every time. You see, for most of us, getting an immediate fix to soothe our emotions, is more persuasive than thinking of the future consequences; we know that washing down a hot dog and fries with a few beers is not so good for our waistline, or our cholesterol, but we do it anyway because it makes us feel good in the moment. To beat emotional eating, you need to take the time to explore yourself to uncover what emotions you may be stuffing down with food.

Keep a Food Diary

One of the best ways to uncover your emotional eating behaviours is by keeping a diary. Food diaries are really telling. Quite often we don't even realise how much, or what, we are eating until it's in black and white. If you write down everything you eat each day it's easy to see where you are going right and where you're going wrong. It will help pick up where you might be eating for emotion instead of hunger, as well as help you learn the calorie content of the foods you eat.

By keeping and reviewing your diaries every week you can start to pick up on recurring patterns. For example, if you can see that you were really busy one day, didn't eat regularly and found yourself starving by dinner time, at which point you overate all the 'wrong' foods, this means you need to be better prepared next week for your busy days. You can then set about a form of action to go grocery shopping to buy lots of convenient foods that you can take with you for the days you don't have time to buy or prepare food.

Diaries can be painful and time consuming to keep but it's an effort that could uncover the necessary answers you're searching for when it comes to losing weight. To really assess your eating habits your Food Diary would ideally consist of:

• What time did I eat?

• What did I eat? (Include specifics, such as serving sizes because two meals that look the same can have extreme differences in their calorie content. For example, did your salad sandwich have

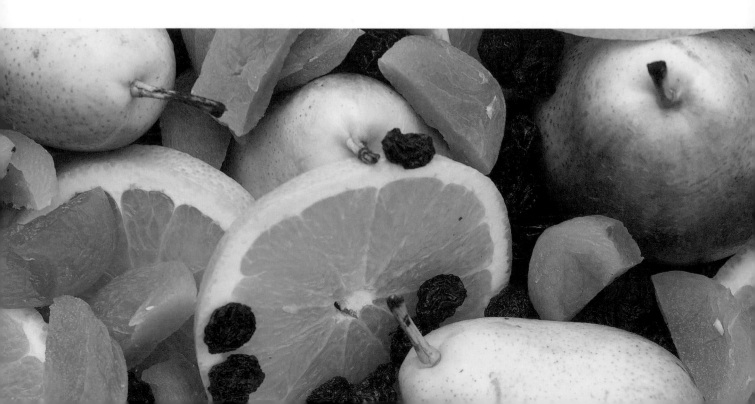

- butter, cheese or mayonnaise? These details can make a huge difference over the course of a week).

- What was I thinking/doing before I ate?

- What was I thinking/doing while I ate?

- Satisfaction/fullness on completion?

Tips for beating emotional eating

When a craving strikes, ask yourself: 'Am I really hungry?' If not, grab a pen and either in your Food Diary (see 'Diaries and planners' in Appendix) or your Weight Loss Journal write down what you're feeling. This will be a positive way to deal with your emotions rather than overeating. It will also help you to get to the bottom of what emotions trigger off your binges.

Find a positive way to nurture yourself and offer comfort—this could be watching a DVD that inspires you or makes you feel good, snuggling up with a hot water bottle and reading a good book, getting outside in the sunshine to sit by a tree, making yourself a nice pot of tea and sitting down in a comfy chair to slowly sip it …What other non-food ways could you give yourself comfort?

- Exercise, do yoga or go for a walk—although this is often the least likely option for most of us, it will make you feel better and less likely to still crave your comfort food post-workout

- Draw yourself a nice warm bath, light some candles and read a magazine

  - Have a massage

  - Get involved in charity work, or simply get more involved in helping your family or friends; when we feed ourselves emotionally, we're less likely to feed ourselves with food

  - Find ways to get excited about healthy eating, such as buying a new recipe book or taking up healthy cooking classes

GREEN TEA CAN HELP RELIEVE SUGAR CRAVINGS AND IS PACKED FULL OF ANTIOXIDANTS.

Susie Burrell

- See a counsellor or psychologist to deal with unresolved issues

- Make a list on your fridge and add to it each day, on what you've done that day to help yourself or others

- Stay busy—if you know you're more inclined to binge at night then organise some night-time exercise or activity to keep you focused

- Stay away from the TV. When you're sitting around you'll be more likely to think about eating.

How much should I eat to lose weight?

While trying to lose weight, men should consume approximately 1500 calories and women 1200 calories each day. Larger people and individuals who exercise heavily may need closer to 1800 calories. Try not to drop your calories too low though as your body needs a certain amount of fuel to maintain your metabolism.

Personalising your diet

In a perfect world, it would be great for everyone to take the time to keep a regular Food Diary, gather information about food and weight loss and learn to adapt an eating program to their individual lifestyle. But, I understand a lot of you don't have the knowledge, find it tedious to keep a Food Diary and feel it's much easier to just follow a set diet. However, if you're really serious about losing weight you are going to need to do some work of your own.

There is no one-size-fits-all diet that suits everyone. You should see a diet as a blueprint. You may have to make accommodations to suit your individual needs and lifestyle. For example, if you're a waiter and work nights, finishing after midnight, you may need to eat more food later in the day to give you energy to get through the night.

You also need to be smart enough to know how to make the right choices when challenging or alternative situations pop up that vary from a designated eating plan.

For example, some diet may tell you that you can't eat a banana at 11 o'clock because the diet plan has a handful of almonds specified for that time. You may have had a really hectic morning and your body is craving a bit of energy—better a banana than a donut!

Tips for personalising a set diet plan:

- If you're really hungry, eat something to tide you over to your next meal! Starvation only exacerbates cravings, making you more likely to break the diet in a big way! Just choose a healthy option: fill up on extra salad, nibble on some unsalted nuts, have a few spoons of yoghurt, spread a little avocado on a slice of natural wholegrain bread. Make it a snack, not another meal—watch portion size.

- Examine what the diet is telling you to eat so you can get knowledge about how to buy a similar meal if you get stuck when you're out.

- If there's a type of food in the plan that you don't like, simply look at the calorie content of that meal and insert something of the same value that you like.

- Meals need to be spaced apart but not too far. You need to find the right eating timetable that suits you and your lifestyle (including work or family commitments).

10. The Eating Guide

So let's roll up our sleeves … it's time to change your eating habits to help you lose weight and put those food issues behind you. To prepare for this, I want you to follow these eight steps:

Ray's eight essential eating steps

Step 1: Go shopping

Remember the burn the boat analogy from Chapter 5? Well, in this case the boat has to be your pantry and fridge. You need to go into the pantry and fridge and burn those boats. You need to grab a big garbage bag and throw out all of the foods that you know are going to hinder your weight loss—I'll give you a hint: all processed packaged foods that don't contain all-natural ingredients!

Next, go shopping and stock up on all fresh ingredients, see Chapter 8 'Understanding food' for the best food choices.

Step 2: Prepare ahead

This is by far the biggest mistake people make when trying to adhere to an eating plan. When you don't get your meals prepared for the day ahead you're setting yourself up for failure. To ensure your success with your weight loss goals, your best weapon is to prepare your meals and snacks in advance:

- Do your grocery shopping every week. You will be surprised how much easier it is to eat healthily when you have a fridge full of variety and healthy foods.

- Buy pre-packaged vegetables that are already washed and cut up.

- Always keep frozen vegetables and fruit in the fridge. They still hold the same nutritional value and save you all the preparation time of washing and cutting.

- Dedicate one night of the week where you put on your favourite TV show or CD, make yourself

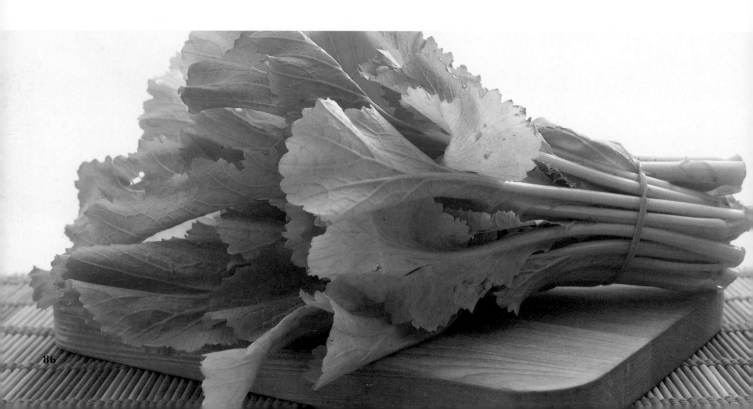

a nice cup of herbal tea or pour yourself a glass of wine. Spend an hour cutting up all of your vegetables and fruit and storing them in the fridge. If you make it an hour of doing something nice to take care of yourself you will enjoy the whole experience and save yourself the hassle of cutting things up when it comes to meal times.

- Think of your day in advance, if you know you'll be really busy, with not much time to eat, take your whole day's worth of food with you.

- Invest in some small containers that carry salad dressing. Take a tin of tuna, a pre-packaged bag of salad, throw it all in and you've got a fast and healthy snack.

- Buy little plastic bags and fill them with a portion of nuts and dried fruit. If you take the whole packet with you you're more likely to scoff down more than you bargained for.

- If you know you're going out for dinner or to a party and you don't want to overeat there, have a light meal before you head out. That way you can just have small snacks over the night without looking like you're dieting or starving yourself.

- When you cook, make extra and freeze it. Convenience is everything when it comes to sticking to a healthy eating plan.

- Stack your fridge with protein-rich snacks such as cold meats, low-fat cheese and yoghurts. When you feel like snacking, having protein rich foods will help stabilise blood sugar levels and control cravings.

Step 3: Spread your meals out

Contrary to popular belief, not all overweight people eat large amounts of food. Sometimes it's actually the practice of skipping meals that causes people to put on weight. There are a couple of problems with this. Firstly, when you skip meals regularly your metabolism slows down. Secondly, when you skip meals then decide to eat when you're starving, you'll usually resort to high sugar or fatty foods to give you that quick fix. It's also these foods that are easy to prepare and are readily available, such as grabbing a packet of chips with dip or melting some cheese on toast.

Ideally, you should be eating three meals and two snacks per day. Breakfast should be within one hour of waking. You can then eat every 2–3 hours.

Step 4: Choose fresh unpackaged foods

Fresh really is best. You might be thinking 'But some natural foods come in packets'. Yes, you're right—some obvious ones are raw nuts, brown rice, skim milk, pre-packaged salad, frozen vegetables, tinned tuna and so on. Aside from the obvious, there are other packaged foods that are okay to eat, but unless you're prepared to become an avid label reader to check for hidden ingredients and additives, you'll have to keep it simple and stick to the 'unpackaged' rule.

Aim to eat most, ideally all, of your food as close to its natural state as possible—that is without being altered or having added ingredients, including sugars, salts, preservatives, colours, flavours, and other additives. A simple rule for choosing your food: Eat foods that grow in the ground, move on the ground or swim in the sea … you just can't go wrong this way!

Step 5: Watch your portion size

Here's a quick and simple guide to gauge correct portions:

Protein: 2–3 serves a day. Serving size: ½ cup lean mince, 100g (3½oz) cooked meat, two small eggs, or 100g (3½oz) of fish. Serving sizes for non-animal protein sources: $1/3$ cup nuts, ¼ cup seeds, ½ cup cooked beans and legumes or a palm size piece of tofu.

Low-fat dairy: 3–4 serves a day. One serve is equal to 1 cup (250ml/8fl oz) low-fat milk, 1 tub (200g/7oz) yoghurt, 2 slices (30g/1oz) reduced-fat cheese.

Wholegrains: 4–5 serves a day. Serving size: A handful—you should be able to hold a handful of carbs, such as brown rice, in your hand, without bits falling out from the sides. Or, no more than 1–2 slices of bread, ½ bread roll, ½ cup cooked porridge, ¼ cup muesli or ½ cup rice or pasta.

Veggies: At least five servings a day.

Fruit: 2 pieces a day.

Fats: 3–4 serves of good fat a day. Add just enough fat for taste or to cook with. Nothing should ever swim in oil. Serving size: $1/8$ avocado, 1 teaspoon olive oil, thin spread of canola spread or all-natural peanut butter, 10–15 nuts or one serve of oily fish.

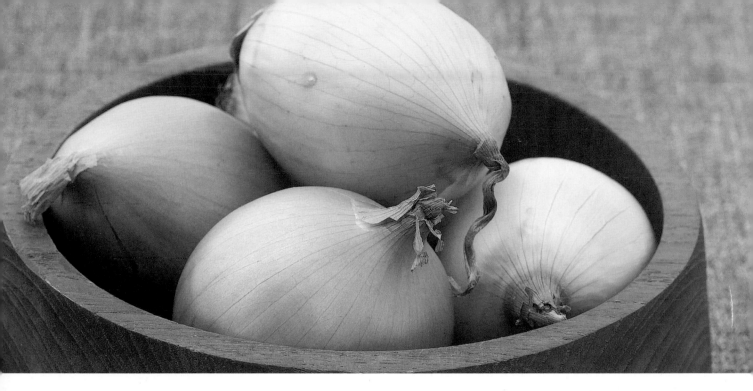

Step 6: Drink water

You need to drink at least two litres of water a day— two litres equates to eight x 250ml (8fl oz) glasses—or enough that your urine is fairly clear. You need extra if you're exercising. Water is essential for weight loss and wellbeing: it prevents dehydration, especially now that we're looking to increase the amount of physical activity you do; helps flush out waste products and replenish your system; cleanses main organs; assists digestion and healthy bowel movements; and keeps everything in working-order. Another water-for-weight-loss advantage is that often we're starving or experiencing out-of-control cravings because we're actually thirsty, not hungry—so you need to keep well hydrated to keep cravings at bay.

Herbal tea, clear broths and water-filled fruit and vegetables also contribute to our daily hydration but should be consumed in addition to your eight or more glasses of water a day.

Note: Soft drinks, juices, alcohol and coffee do not count for water. Be mindful of the fact that caffeine and alcohol dehydrate you so be sure to have one glass of water for every cup of coffee, caffeinated soft drink or alcoholic beverage to balance it out. Also, many people might think they don't eat that much but on looking at their diets are consuming more calories from beverages than they realise—such as hidden sugars in soft drinks, some sports drinks and flavoured water, and cordials; high calorie content of some juices and smoothies bought from juice bars; and hidden fats and sugars in daily coffee purchases with added extras such as cream, chocolate flakes and flavourings. Why drink your calories when you can eat them?

Step 7: Be mindful of your eating habits

From this day forward, you need to be present while you eat. This means, turn off the TV, stop work, step away from your computer, put down the phone. If your mind is on other things when you eat, it's too easy to lose track of how many times your hand has dipped into a bag of chips or that you're actually full, even though you're on your second serving. Take the time and focus on the food you're eating; you'll appreciate it more this way.

And remember to be mindful of emotional eating. Food only has one real purpose: to give us fuel to function, in the same way we fuel our cars to drive. Eating for any other reason—depression, stress, boredom and so on—gets you into trouble. Stop yourself before every meal and ask, 'Am I really hungry?' If not, ask 'What am I really hungry for?' Perhaps it's company because you're feeling lonely, comfort because you feel down, relaxation because you feel stressed. Take the time to know what you're really feeling and use non-food ways to respond to your feelings. Like any habit, it will take time to create a new way of dealing with your emotions, but practice makes perfect!

Step 8: Regularly review your Food Diary

Don't expect your eating habits to change overnight or to get things right every time. You're going to make mistakes, fall off the wagon, want to give up, give up, and start all over again. Like a learned skill, you need to unlearn your old eating behaviours and re-learn a new way of eating. This won't be easy at first, because you probably have a lot to learn. By keeping your Food Diary you can fast track the learning process by seeing where things are working and where things are not. This is crucial for fine tuning your diet, and making the necessary changes to move closer to your weight loss goals—

for example, by regularly looking over your Food Diary you might pick up where you ate for comfort instead of hunger or where you could have made better food choices or work out where you can best cut calories because your weight loss has hit a plateau. Remember, learning how to lose weight and maintain your weight loss is always a work in progress!

Choosing your eating plan

There are two approaches for you to choose from: the 500-calorie-cutting Plan and my special 4 Stage eating plan.

Both Chris and Adro ate around 1200 calories per day. However, everyone is different: heavier people, those with a lot of weight to lose, and more active people have a higher calorie requirement. And if you're currently consuming a lot of calories (most likely if you're overweight), jumping to a

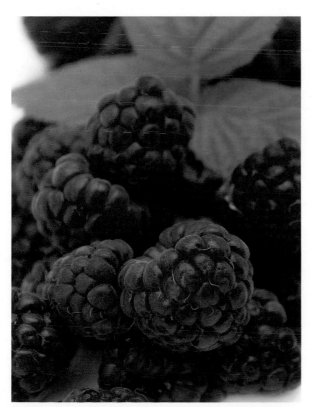

1200-calorie eating plan may be too hard to stick to. Also, not everyone wants to follow a set diet plan, preferring to incorporate their own favourite foods and meals into their own diet plan. The point being: there is no one-size-fits-all eating plan. You have to find an approach that works for you. To help you in this process you can choose from the 500-calorie-cutting plan or my 4 Stage eating plan.

Choose the 500-calorie-cutting plan if you want flexibility in your eating plan, don't mind doing the hard work of counting calories and making your own food choices, and would prefer to make slow and gradual changes, at your own pace.

Choose my 4 Stage eating plan if you find counting calories a bit of a pain, and would prefer having the guesswork taken out.

The 500-calorie-cutting Plan

You need to make a caloric deficit of around 500 calories a day to lose half a kilogram (one pound) per week. Probably the most flexible and achievable method, especially for those starting out, is to simply subtract 500 calories from your current calorie intake. The main benefits of this approach are:

- You don't have to cut everything out all at once, which means it will be much more enjoyable, realistic and sustainable.

- The more you weigh the greater the need for calories; so a generic 1500-calorie diet for an obese person as opposed to a slightly overweight person means the heavier person would have to cut more calories and feel much more deprived!

- You don't have to do the equations to find out your calorie requirements. Just write down what you're eating each day (see sample next page), decrease your daily calories from there, as well as increase your exercise, and you will lose weight.

- You slowly wean yourself off the high calories.

Step 1: Keep a log of your food intake for the next seven days in the Calorie Cutting Planner in Appendix (or simply make your own template on your computer or in your Weight Loss Journal). Be specific, including serving sizes, calories and 'hidden' ingredients such as a tablespoon of oil in a stir-fry. Source these in a pocket calorie counting book (a must-have for those wanting to lose weight) or by visiting *www.calorieking.com*.

Step 2: Add up the total amount of calories you average per day (add up the total calories you eat for the week and divide by 7 to get the average).

Step 3: Look over your diet, and make a list of things you can cut out to reduce 500 calories each day, or simply cross them off your daily plan.

Step 4: Repeat steps 1–3 when your weight loss plateaus.

My list of 500-calorie reductions

Hold the butter on your morning toast, skip your morning biscuit while still enjoying your afternoon cookie, have strawberries for dessert on their own and take your coffee and tea without sugar and save 508 calories.

Sample calorie cutting planner

Day: Monday

Time	Description	Size	Calories
7am	Fruit loaf	2 thin slices	161
	~~Butter~~	~~2 tsp~~	~~72~~
10am	Takeaway latte with full-fat milk	Large	224
	~~Sugar~~	~~2 tsp~~	~~40~~
	~~Shortbread~~	~~1 biscuit~~	~~86~~
11am	Apple	1 medium	78
12pm	Subway chicken fillet sandwich (no dressing, oil or cheese)	6-inch sub	297
3pm	Choc-chip cookie	1 medium	59
	Tea with full-fat milk	1 cup	23
	~~Sugar~~	~~1 tsp~~	~~20~~
7pm	2 grilled lean pork chops	200g (71/4 oz)	380
	Potato salad with mayonnaise	1 cup	360
	Cup of tea with full-fat milk	30ml milk	20
8pm	~~Ice cream~~	~~3 regular scoops~~	~~290~~
	Strawberries	5 small	25
		Total:	**~~2135~~ 1627**

The Eating Plans

Ray Kelly's 4 Stage Eating Plan

This is the meal plan that has brought about massive transformations on people all over Australia. On this meal plan most people will average a weight loss of 1.5kg-2kg per week. But please remember, if you make changes to it then you could dilute your results!

Overview

Stage 1 - Detox

In Stage 1 you will become detoxed from all the sugars, fats and salts. You're eating a lot of fresh, unprocessed foods, primarily meat and vegetables or salad.

This should be followed for at least 2 weeks, but I'd advise that you follow it as long as you can.

This is the Stage where you will see the fastest results so the longer you stay on Stage 1 the faster you will reach your goal weight.

Everyone 'slips up' along the way (but obviously the less you slip up the greater your results) and that can be the difference between being successful at weight-loss or not, so this is the eating plan you need to come back to if you stumble while on the other stages.

You may find this meal plan a bit bland but I make no apology for that. This stage consists of REAL food. This is what REAL food tastes like, before all of the salt, sugar and fats are added. The

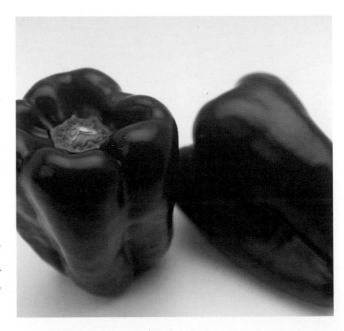

problem is we've become so accustomed to processed foods that our tastes now crave sugary, salty and fatty foods, yet our tolerance for them have increased, so we require so much more to gain the same satisfaction. And our bodies are suffering! Just look at the statistics on weight-related illnesses such as Type 2 diabetes and heart disease. Complications from these issues are hospitalising and killing people at a growing rate right around the world. In most cases, this can be avoided simply by consuming a diet predominantly consisting of fresh foods and walking each day.

Stage 2 - Introduction of more variety

Once you've lost 10 percent of your body weight you can move on to Stage 2. In this stage, you get to introduce some of the other recipes we provide. This is so that you still keep to eating clean fresh foods, but have the chance to gain more variety at mealtime.

Stage 3 - Introduction of your own foods

If you are to lose weight and keep it off it's important that I teach you how to introduce the style of foods you like. Once you are within 10kg of your goal weight you can move to Stage 3. In this stage you get to introduce the recipes you like. By now you would have learnt a lot about how various foods, and portions affect your body, so you'll find you'll be able to make smart choices.

Stage 4 - Maintenance

Stage 4 is the Maintenance Phase. Many people struggle to keep their weight off. But I've made it as simple as it can be. You get to eat whatever you like, and exercise as often as you like.

Sounds good right?

There are just 2 simple rules. You can read all about them later in this chapter!

Stage 1

How to make sure you succeed

I can help you lose all the weight you want to, but we need to get one thing clear. You have tried your way and it didn't work so if you're serious about it this time you have to follow everything I say and follow it to the letter. If you try to adjust it to what you like or don't like then this will be just another weight loss attempt added to your list and you'll be in the same boat this time next year.

I will provide you with an itemised meal plan so it is very easy to follow. For best results you need to follow it exactly how it is written. Initially you will be asking yourself 'I wonder if I can have this?' or 'I wonder if I can have that?' but it's all quite simple, if it's not written on the meal plan page then it's just not in the program! Easy right?

So here's the plan!

The Stage 1 meal plan will see you detox your body and reduce your cravings for sweet, salty, and fatty foods. Remember, if you sneak these foods in you're just feeding the cravings!

This meal plan may seem a little extreme to some but it is all just fresh foods. The kind of foods our bodies were meant to eat and the type of foods our ancestors ate for their whole life. We have grown so accustomed to smothering our foods with salty, fatty or sweet ingredients that this is the taste we now look for in our foods. The problem is this is the cause of most of our illness (and medications!) as we age. One thing I will say though is that most people will lose between 3–5 kg in this first week, so give me 7 days and see how you feel about the food then!

Just remember though you don't have to eat like this forever. We give you more variety as we go and the end goal is to have you eating the kinds of foods you do enjoy, just in a more balanced way. I'll show you how to introduce the foods as we go!

I need you to eat fresh foods and try to have something every few hours. For example, if you eat breakfast at 8am, have a snack at 10:30, lunch at 1pm, a snack at 4pm, and dinner at 7pm. For fastest results, try to keep your meals and snacks higher in protein. Eating this way will also keep you fuller for longer. Just remember, you need to watch how much you eat in each meal too, because you can still put on weight if you eat too many healthy foods.

As I mentioned previously, if it's not written in black and white in the following meal plan then you can't have it. However, just to make things clear I'd like to highlight some of the foods that are to be totally avoided (just for now, they all come back in down the track). You cannot have cheese, rice, pasta, potato, salad dressings, sauces, oil, salt, or desserts. (These are some of the main foods that will blow out your calories/fluid levels).

Here are some important rules:

- All weights given for meats and vegetables are 'raw weights'.

- All meats are to be grilled or BBQ'd. Fish can also be either poached or baked in foil.

- Fruit options for Stage 1 are apple, orange, banana, 250g strawberries, 100g blueberries, peach, pear or mandarin.

- Either salad or vegetables can be had at lunch or dinner (see the meal plan for selections and portions).

- You can cook with fresh chilli, garlic, or ginger, but nothing in a jar or tube (it has to be fresh!).

- You can use fresh herbs—nothing dried or in a shaker.

- You can have 2 coffees per day, but no lattes, cappuccinos, flat whites, etc. Simply a black coffee with a splash of milk. You cannot have any sweetener, sugar or honey. It is shown to increase your cravings and that is not something we need for you right now!

- You can also have 6 cups of tea a day, more if you are having green tea.

- If you like eating late at night, divide your dinner into 2 portions and have one serving at 7pm and another at 9pm.

Here is a the meal plan:

BREAKFAST	SNACK	LUNCH	SNACK	DINNER
3 weet-bix with 250 ml of skim milk (no sugar, sweetener, honey, or fruit) Or 2/3 cup of rolled oats with 250 ml of skim milk (no sugar, sweetener, honey, or fruit) Or 2 boiled or poached eggs and 1 piece of toast (small scraping of butter)	1 piece of fruit, or a 95 g can of tuna in springwater	Tuna (95 g, in springwater) and salad or vegetables (see below for contents of salad and vegetables) Or 2 x eggs and salad or vegetables (see below for contents of salad and vegetables) Or Chicken (150 g of breast meat only) and salad or vegetables (see below for contents of salad and vegetables) Or 8 King prawns (jumbo shrimp) and salad or vegetables (see below for contents of salad and vegetables)	1 x piece of fruit, or 95 g can of tuna in springwater	1. Steak (200 g) and vegetables or salad 2. Fresh white fish (300 g) and vegetables or salad 3. Chicken (300 g) and vegetables or salad 4. 15 x King prawns (jumbo shrimp) and vegetables or salad *Salad consists of:* 1/2 tomato 1/4 onion 1/2 carrot 4 mushrooms 1/2 capsicum 50 g (handful) baby spinach/lettuce Optional sprinkle of pepper (no salt) *Dressing:* **Juice of 1/2 lemon squeezed over the top, or 1 tablespoon balsamic vinegar** *Vegetables consist of:* 6 x broccoli florets ½ x zucchini 2 x pieces of pumpkin (50 g each) 10 x beans

If there is anything in the vegetables you do not like, then you can swap with one of the following:

6 cauliflower florets

1 cup cabbage

1 cup spinach

1 button squash

3 Brussel sprouts

Note: Winter Choices

When the weather gets a little colder it's great to be eating the warmer foods and soup is a good choice. The problem is that it is usually very high in sodium which will affect your weight on the scales as well as your blood pressure. So you need to make the soup yourself. However, most soup stocks sold in supermarkets are very high in salt (even the ones branded 'salt reduced'!) so you will need to make your stock yourself. This can be done by adding some carrots, celery, onion and some chicken carcasses to a pot of water and simmering it over a few hours. Be sure to drain the stock before use.

Stage 2

Once you've lost 10 percent of your body weight you have the choice of moving on to Stage 2. However, the fastest weight loss will occur in Stage 1 so if you have quite a bit to lose and you don't mind that style of eating then stay on Stage 1.

On Stage 2 you can start to introduce some more variety in the form of the recipes provided in this book (See Michael Moore's recipes later on page 105). You can also add in stir-fries. Just make sure that you're not using sauces that are high in salt or sugar (unfortunately, most are). My favourites are balsamic vinegar or ketjup manis (this is sweet Indonesian soy sauce and is available in most supermarkets).

While on this stage, if there is ever a week where you don't lose weight then I want you to move back to Stage 1 (as we know you will definitely keep losing weight there).

General food changes for Stage 2

200 g lean lamb steak, or 200 g lean pork steak can now be added to your meat options at night. They must be lean steaks though and not chops, cutlets or roasts.

1 x small boiled potato (not chips or mashed potato) or half a cob of corn can be added to your vegetable options, so long as they are eaten in a meal that contains meat

The following spices can now be used: paprika, cumin, tumeric, curry (just be sure that each of these are not high in sodium!)

Dressing 1: Yoghurt Dressing
60 g fat-free natural yoghurt
1 tablespoon olive oil
black pepper

Dressing 2: Lemon and Honey Dressing
2 tablespoons (120 ml) lemon juice
½ tablespoon minced lemon peel
¼ cup extra virgin olive oil
2 tablespoons vinegar
½ teaspoon oregano
½ tablespoon honey
A pinch of black pepper

For each of these dressings, one serve is one tablespoon.

A salsa can be added to your meals if you reduce your meat portion by 50 g.

Salsa 1:

1 medium tomato, diced
1 small onion, finely chopped
½ fresh jalapeno pepper, seeded and chopped
2 sprigs fresh coriander, finely chopped
1 onion, finely chopped
⅛ teaspoon pepper
Serves 4

Salsa 2:

1 ripe tomato, diced
½ capsicum, diced
1 white onion, diced
½ bunch fresh coriander, for garnish
1 tablespoon fresh lemon juice
Serves 2

Stage 3

You can move to Stage 3 once you are within 10 kg of your goal weight. If you are to keep the weight off then it's important that you learn how to re-introduce the foods you like and Stage 3 is where you get to put what you've learnt so far into action.

Here's some tips for adding new foods in:

To begin with, just change a few of your night time meals.

See how your body responds at your weekly weigh in and if you keep losing weight, change some more meals.

If you didn't lose as much weight as you had hoped for then either reduce the portion size of the new meals or change them altogether.

11. Recipes

Michael Moore is an experienced and respected chef, starting out in some of London's best restaurants. Now 26 years into a career spanning two continents, Michael has owned and managed numerous top restaurants in both London and Sydney including The Ritz Hotel London, Kables, Craigend, Hotel Nikko, The Bluebird London, Bennelong, Prunier's, Bonne Femme and Wildfire. Michael has earned critical appraise on both sides of the globe, as well as a number of coveted media awards. Michael has appeared on television for the last seven years and is currently the chef and owner of O Bar and Dining in Sydney. *Blood Sugar: The Family* is Michael's third book, and follows *Moore to Food and Blood Sugar.*

Note: These recipes are allowed in to your meal plan exactly as they are. Just because an ingredient is in one of these recipes it doesn't mean you can use it in other recipes.

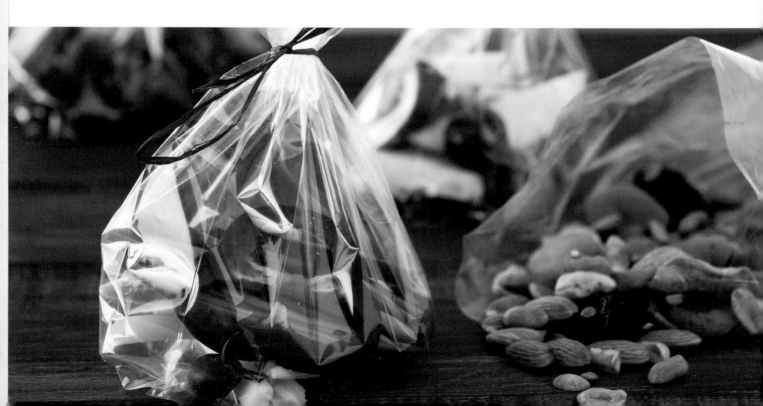

Pack 'n Go Snack Bags

Giant trail mix

pepitas/pumpkin seeds
raw cashew nuts
raw peanuts
dried apples
dried apricots
dried prunes
whole almonds

Roast the pepitas, cashew nuts and peanuts in a 360°F/180°C oven for 12 minutes, and allow to cool before placing in the bags. Mix your preferred selection of remaining ingredients, making sure to include plenty of seeds and nuts.

Crispy salad bags

celery sticks
baby cherry tomatoes
baby corn cobs
sliced red peppers/capsicums
carrot sticks
green beans

Wash and dry the figs, cut the mango cheeks, leaving the skin on and slice a criss-cross into the flesh with a small knife. When they are ready to eat, invert the slices to eat each small square at a time. Leave the stones in the cherries and also leave the skin on the pineapple slices, it will keep fresh.

Tropical fruit treats

sliced fresh pineapple
sliced fresh mango
black figs
red cherries

Wash and dry all the berries, handling them carefully as they are fragile. Change the berries to whatever is in season, and keep as chilled as possible. Berries are high in fibre but also sugar, so keep portion sizes small.

Protein boost, scrambled eggs with tomatoes

8 ripe Roma tomatoes
pepper
1 clove fresh garlic, crushed
1 medium red chilli, finely chopped
½ teaspoon superfine/caster sugar
8 large eggs
4 egg whites
3oz (80g) silken tofu
2 tablespoons olive oil
½ bunch fresh basil
grainy bread, toasted, to serve

1. Preheat oven to 300°F/180°C. Halve the tomatoes lengthways and place onto a baking tray. Brush with half the olive oil, then season with pepper.

2. Spread tomatoes with the crushed garlic and chopped chilli, then dust lightly with caster sugar.

3. Place onto a tray and roast in oven for 25–35 minutes.

4. Meanwhile, in a mixing bowl place the whole eggs, egg whites and tofu; whisk well together and season with pepper.

5. Heat a medium-sized non-stick frying pan over a high heat, add the remaining olive oil. Add the fresh basil leaves and cook for 10 seconds. Add the eggs and tofu mixture, leave to cook for 10 seconds without stirring and, using chopsticks or a wooden spoon, gradually stir the eggs from the outside of the pan to the centre.

6. Once eggs and tofu become creamy, remove from the heat. The scrambled eggs should be undercooked and slightly liquid, however, the eggs will continue to cook in the pan. Serve on grainy toasted bread with the roasted tomatoes.

Serves 4

In consultation with Michael Moore, salt has been removed from this recipe.

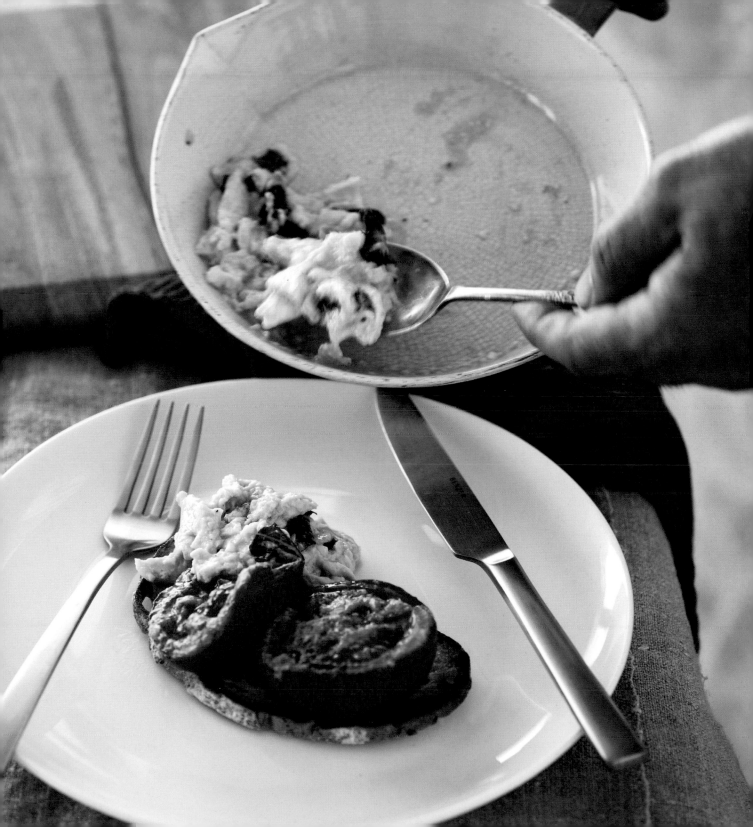

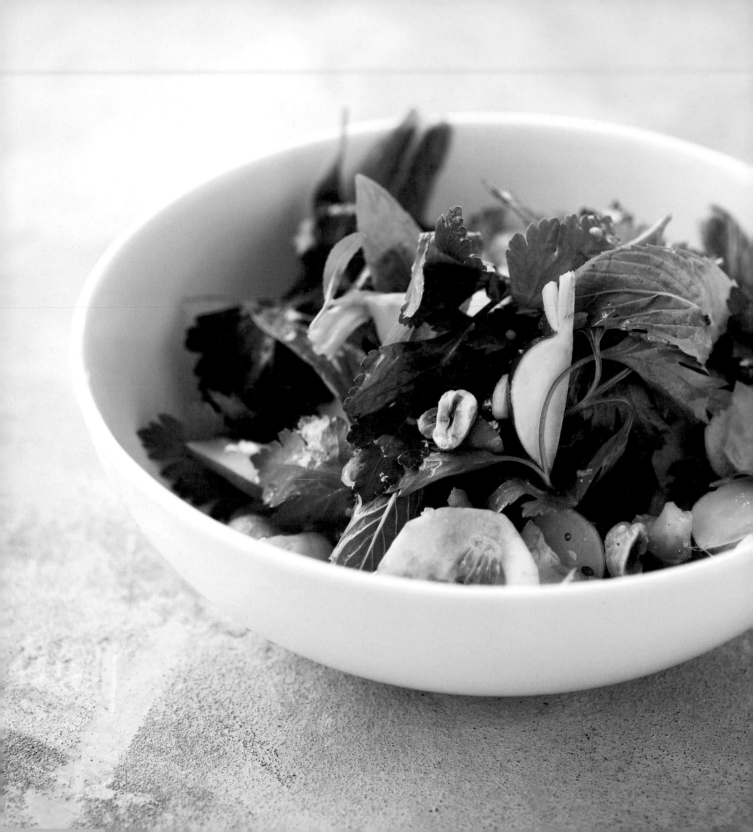

Cucumber salad with pear & citrus dressing

2 cucumbers, sliced and peeled
1 lime
1 tablespoon hazelnuts
1 tablespoon macadamia nuts
1 bunch red radishes, quartered
1 bunch continental parsley
1 ripe pear, thinly sliced
1 bunch mint
½ bunch cilantro/coriander leaves
pinch pepper

Dressing
½ teaspoon yellow mustard seeds
1 tablespoon orange juice
1 tablespoon olive oil

1. Using a vegetable peeler, remove skin from cucumber. Using a mandolin, slice thinly into a bowl. Squeeze the juice of the lime over and leave to stand in the fridge for an hour to soften.

2. Preheat a small frying pan and dry roast the hazelnuts and macadamia nuts for approximately 3–5 minutes until they go light brown. Allow to cool and roughly chop.

3. In a larger bowl, place coriander and mint leaves, radish quarters, thinly sliced pears and the toasted nuts. Add sliced cucumbers.

4. Place dressing ingredients in a small jar and shake well. Pour the dressing over the salad, mix and serve.

Serves 4

In consultation with Michael Moore, salt has been removed from this recipe.

Sweet chicken skewers

8 bamboo skewers
2 large chicken breasts
2 tablespoons agave nectar
3 tablespoons light soy sauce
juice and zest of one lemon
small knob of fresh ginger, grated
sesame seeds and fresh herbs, to serve

1. Soak the bamboo skewers in cold water for 30 minutes. Cut the chicken breast into small strips.

2. Combine all other ingredients in a small bowl. Thread the chicken strips onto the skewers and brush with the marinade mixture. Cook on a hot barbecue plate or in a non-stick frying pan. Don't keep turning but allow skewers to caramelise and even char on the edges, this should only take approximately 5–6 minutes to cook.

3. Sprinkle with some sesame seeds and fresh herbs.

Serves 4

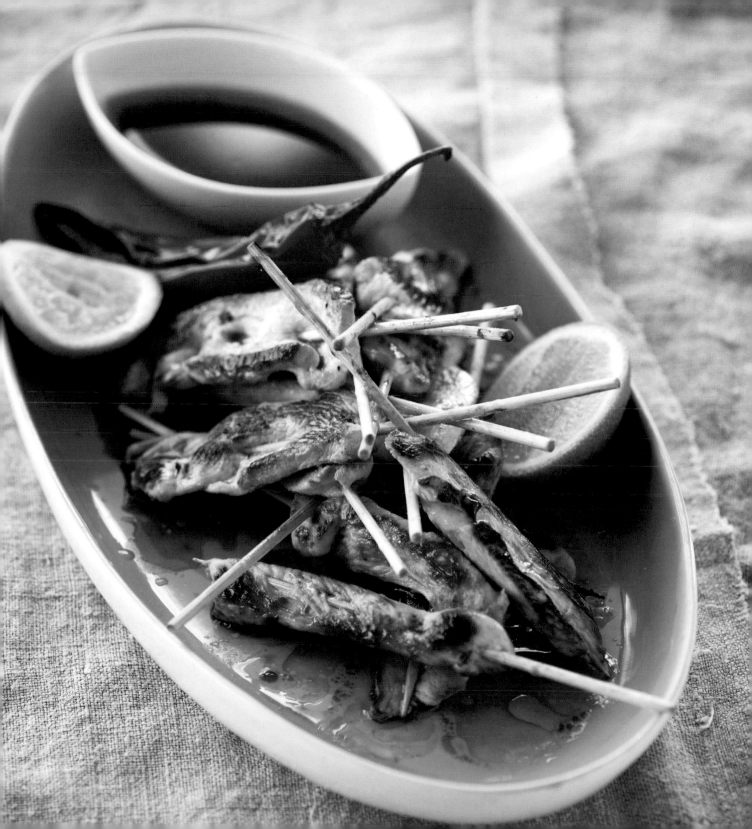

Barbecue rib steak with fresh horseradish & chilli

4 x 12oz (300g) rib eye steaks on the bone
1 tablespoon olive oil
pepper
2oz (60g) piece of fresh horseradish
1 cup red mustard or red frill leaves
½ cup pickled chilli

1. Preheat a barbecue plate or skillet pan.

2. Rub the steaks with a little olive oil and season with pepper. Place the steaks onto the hot grill plate and cook to your liking. Remove from the grill plate and allow the steaks to rest for 2 minutes before serving them.

3. Slice the beef onto the plate. Sprinkle the red frill leaves and loosely scatter the pickled chilli salsa over as well. Finally using a microplane-style grater, grate the fresh horseradish on the top.

Serves 4

In consultation with Michael Moore, salt has been removed from this recipe.

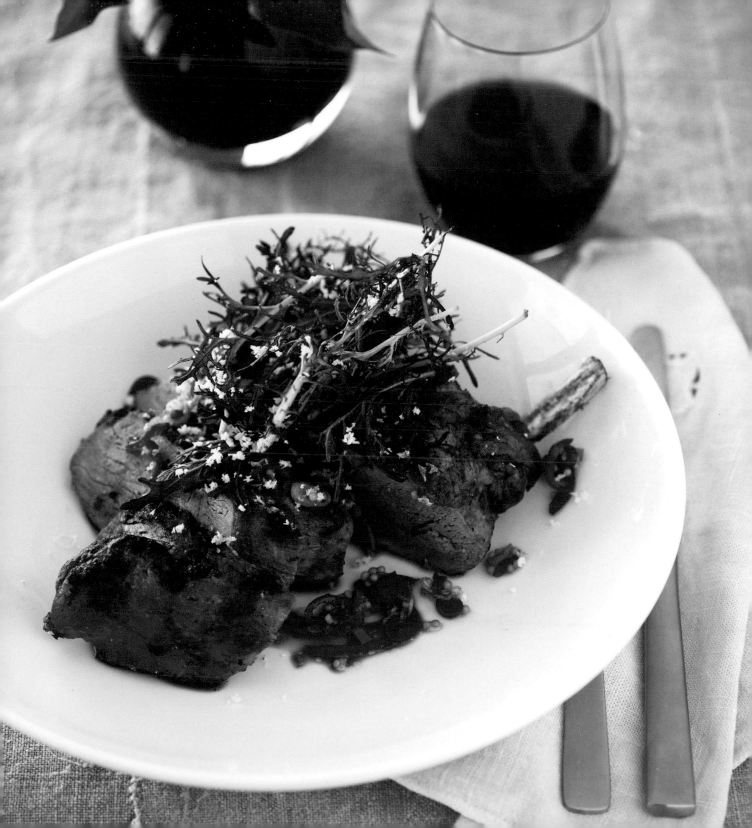

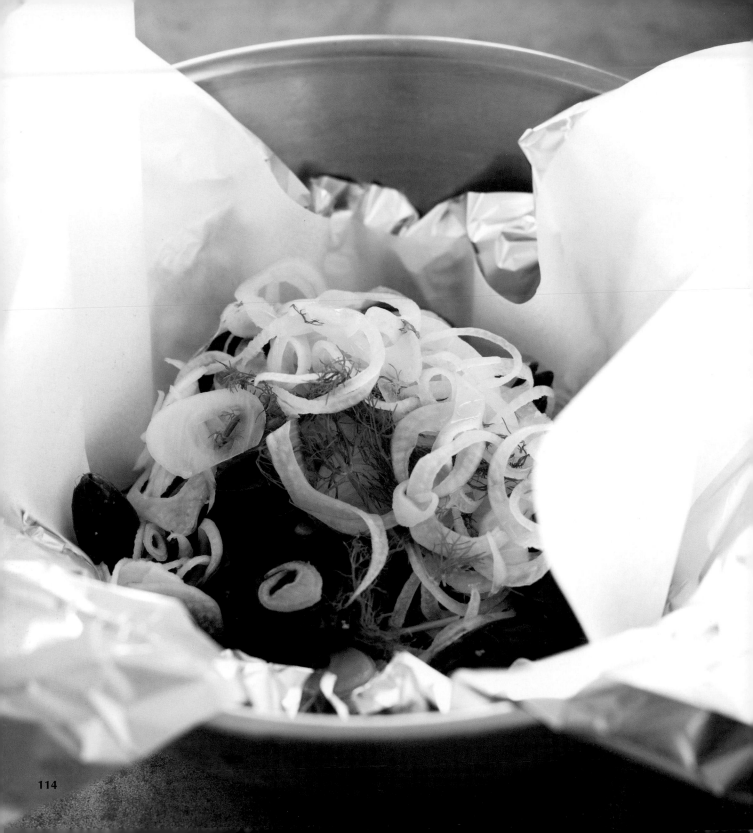

Steamed mussels in a bag with fennel

1 onion, finely sliced
1 fennel bulb, finely sliced
2lb (1kg) live black mussels
2 fresh bay leaves
1 clove garlic
fresh black pepper
½ glass white wine
½ bunch dill or fennel tips

1. Preheat the oven to 360°F/180°C. Place the sliced onions and fennel into a small saucepan full of water and bring to the boil. Rinse under cold water and drain.

2. Wash and clean the mussels making sure all of the small beards and any barnacles have been removed. Lay a large sheet of aluminium foil on a bench and cover with a piece of greaseproof paper of similar size. Place the foil and paper sheets over a bowl or colander and push down in the middle to form a bowl shape.

3. Place mussels, blanched fennel, onions, fresh bay leaves, garlic and a few black peppercorns into the foil and paper then pour in wine.

4. Using both hands, draw the side together to form a bag and twist the top to seal the bag, tie with a piece of butchers twine.

5. Place bag into the oven for 15 minutes. The mussels will steam open and form a light sauce.

6. Open the bag at the table and sprinkle the dill tips on the top and serve with some finger bowls and hot bread or sweet potato chips.

Serves 4

Chinese cabbage & chicken salad

1 Chinese cabbage/wombok
2 sticks of celery
4 red radishes, finely sliced
1 red apple
4oz (120g) roast chicken breast
½ cup low-fat cheddar cheese, grated

Dressing
2 tablespoons light olive oil
1 teaspoon of white wine vinegar
1 teaspoon light soy sauce
1 small knob fresh ginger,grated
1 tablespoon currants
pepper

1. Wash and dry the Chinese cabbage and peel the celery. Using a sharp knife or a mandolin, cut them both as fine as possible. Place into a mixing bowl with the radishes.

2. Quarter and core the apple and slice finely. Tear the chicken breast into small pieces, then mix it and the cheese into the salad.

3. Place all of the dressing ingredients into a small jar with a lid and shake well. Pour over the salad, mix through, and serve.

Serves 4

In consultation with Michael Moore, salt has been removed from this recipe.

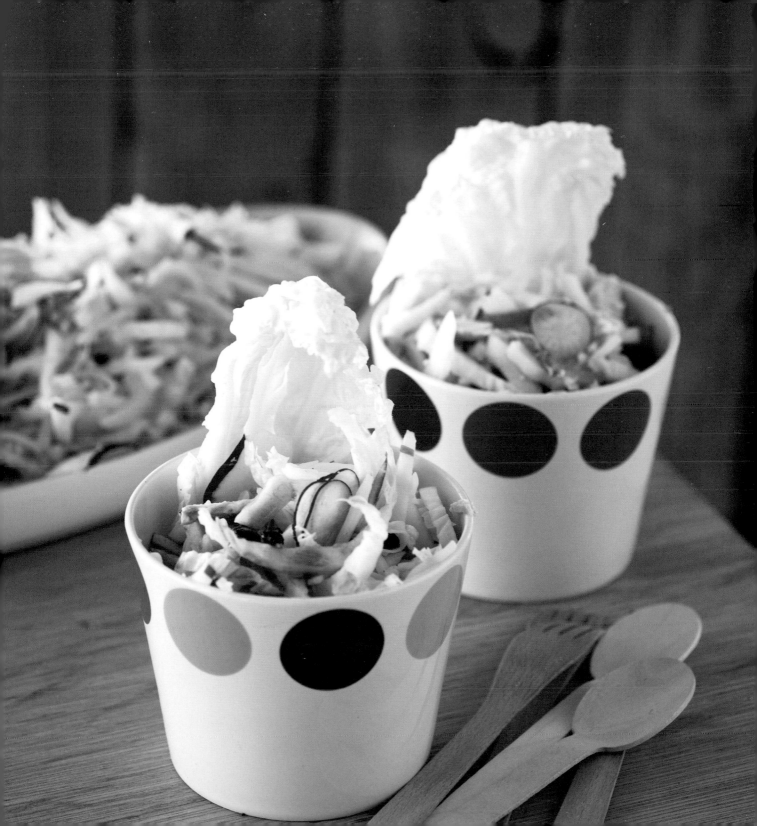

PART THREE: TRAINING LIKE A WINNER

The final step in your journey to being a winner is exercise! Combined with the right mind-set and eating plan, which you have hopefully gained from working through the book so far, exercise will seal the deal on your weight loss. Whether you can't stand the thought of exercise or you currently work out, there are tips to make sure exercise and activity works to your weight loss advantage. I can't sum up the importance of physical activity for weight loss any better than one of the visitors on my online forum when she said: 'Now I must live my life feet first, not teeth first.'

START A WALKING GROUP! IT'S MORE SOCIAL AND YOU ALL GET TO FEED OFF EACH OTHER'S MOTIVATION.

Ray Kelly

12. Move it to lose it

Exercise plays an important role in weight loss: by burning extra calories we can achieve our goals much faster. But exercise is much more important than this. It can increase the strength in our heart, lungs, and muscles; increase the range of motion in our joints; and can even improve our immune system. And the benefits are not just physical. Regular exercise can also make you feel better mentally, increasing your self-esteem and even improving your ability to concentrate. Basically, exercise is your golden ticket to an easier life—you'll get up each morning with more 'spring' in your step, you'll do day-to-day activities with ease such as shopping, cleaning the house and running after your kids, and finish the day with some sounder sleeping.

Weight loss is just one positive side effect of exercise. Many people become disheartened if they don't lose a lot of weight, or any weight, after undertaking an exercise program. This is a mistake. Even if you don't have a loss on the scales, you will most definitely experience improvement in your health and how you feel. There are many convincing reasons to make exercise as much of a habit as brushing your teeth, including the following:

- Reduction in total cholesterol: decrease in low-density lipoprotein (LDL) cholesterol (the bad stuff) and an increase in high-density lipoprotein (HDL) cholesterol (the good stuff)

- Improved insulin sensitivity

- Improved blood glucose levels

- Reduced risk of developing type 2 diabetes

- Stress management

- Boosted metabolism

- Increased energy and libido

- Improved flexibility, strength, coordination and balance, reducing the risk of injury

- Higher self-esteem

- Reduced likelihood of anxiety and depression

- Natural anti-depressant: research has shown regular, moderate exercise to be as effective as medication in combating depression

- Reduced risk of cardiovascular disease, stroke, high blood pressure, osteoporosis and some cancers.

Cancer

The World Health Organisation (WHO) estimates that up to one-third of cancers of the colon, kidney and digestive tract are caused by being overweight and inactive.

Getting active

Exercise is different to 'activity'. Exercise involves doing a dedicated workout for a set period of time. Put on your sneakers and workout clothes and head out for a power walk or run and you've exercised. Head to the gym for an aerobics class and you've exercised. Lace up your gloves and get stuck into the punching bag and you've exercised. Play a game of soccer and you've exercised. Get the drift?

Activity, on the other hand, refers to everyday occurrences that require you to move your body with a little exertion—everything from walking around to do the groceries, to scrubbing the bathroom, to sweeping the floor. It's incidental exercise; you didn't necessarily plan to do it but you 'accidentally' got some exercise benefits from your day-to-day activities and chores. Increase your activity by:

- Whenever you have the opportunity, use walking as your method of transportation

- Take the stairs instead of lifts or escalators; if you already take the stairs, take them two at a time

- Include the kids in your exercise time; you could push them in the stroller, or play 'moving' games

- Grab your coffee takeaway and meet your friend for a walk-and-talk

- Go for a morning weekend walk to your favourite local café and have a healthy breakfast

- Take regular breaks throughout your work day. Include a short walk in this time and you'll be surprised how mentally refreshed you'll be; studies have shown that you'll be much more productive as well

- Get up and get your own coffee, lunch or paperwork instead of having others bring it to you

- Get off the bus or train one stop early and walk the extra distance

- Do away with labour-saving devices such as the remote control, clothes dryer and dishwasher and do all the chores yourself

- Ditch the hired help, do the housework and gardening yourself

- Park as far away from the shop entrance as possible

- Walk the dog, or a neighbour's dog, each day

- Walk the kids to school instead of driving them

- Buy a pedometer and work towards reaching a target of 10 000 steps per day

- Sweep the carpet with a straw broom, rather than vacuuming, or wear a weighted backpack as you sweep or vacuum.

3 levels of activity

Health authorities around the world encourage us to be more active, include at least 30 minutes of moderate activity most days and incorporate more vigorous activity for extra health and fitness.

Risk factor

Physical inactivity is one of the biggest risk factors for ill health and disease.

First, be more active

Our bodies were designed to move—to walk, run, jump, bend and so on—because back in the early times we had to be movers in order to survive, to do things like find food and build shelter. Any opportunity to move your body and be active is what your body craves. Sitting and sleeping for long periods of time and letting technology do our chores for us is unhealthy. See any chance to move—everything from getting up off the couch to change the channel to walking to buy the newspaper to playing with your kids—as a chance to keep moving your body the way nature intended.

Secondly, include at least 30 minutes of moderate-intensity physical activity most days

Iron some clothes, sweep the floor or stroll around the shops and you probably don't get out of breath. Take on some slightly harder activities, such as scrubbing mould off tiles or pulling out some stubborn weeds or walking briskly and you probably feel your heart beating a little harder and your rate of breathing a little faster. This is working at a moderate intensity; your heart and breathing is slightly elevated, so you could talk while you were doing the activity but not sing. Also, you might like to know that research has shown that accumulating short bouts of moderate-intensity activity, of at least 10 minutes each time, can be just as effective for your health. So you can accumulate small bouts of 10–15 minutes of continuous activity—such as a 10-minute brisk walk to the bus stop in the morning, a 10-minute walk in your lunchbreak, and a 10-minute walk after dinner with the family— or you can do 30 minutes all at once, such as cycling to work at a medium pace, or digging in the garden.

Finally, add more vigorous intensity activity for extra health and fitness

Go for a power walk or jog and you'll be huffing and puffing, finding it hard to complete a full sentence in between breaths, and you're likely to have worked up a bit of a sweat. This is working at a vigorous intensity and is what you experience when you exercise or play sports such as football or basketball. This type of activity can be added, not substituted for, the everyday activity you do, for those looking for extra health and fitness benefits. For best results, you need to do this type of activity for a minimum of 30 minutes at least three to four times a week.

The next step: Exercise

While incorporating more movement and 30 minutes of moderate activity most days of the week is great for kick-starting your weight loss and gaining health benefits, to really get greater fitness and weight loss you need to do dedicated weekly workouts. By including actual 'exercise' in your life you will gain added health and fitness benefits:

- Extra protection against heart disease
- Extra calorie burning

- Planned exercise sessions give you the ability to burn more calories in a shorter period of time

- Exercise can be more social than incidental activity, such as playing team sports or doing an exercise class

- Planned exercise sessions usually entail following a structured program whereas incidental activity does not, which means that you're less likely to shorten the duration or reduce the intensity when exercising.

A well-balanced exercise program covers three cornerstones of fitness: strength, stamina and suppleness. Strength relates to being strong in your muscles, bones and joints. To do this you need to do resistance training. Stamina means building your cardiovascular fitness. To do this you need to do aerobic exercise, most commonly referred to as cardio exercise. Suppleness relates to your flexibility. To get flexible you need to stretch. This means a workout program needs to contain resistance training, cardio training and stretching. Let's look at each of these in a bit more detail.

Resistance training—for strength

Resistance training—also called strength or weight-training—involves more than lifting your humble dumbbell. Resistance training is doing any exercise where the muscles oppose a force. What's the source of this force? It can be your own body weight, water, immovable objects, free weights, weight machines, resistance bands or another person.

Tools of the trade

Some common examples of resistance training equipment:

- Barbell

- Dumbbells

- Medicine ball

- Resistance band

- Ankle weights

- Weighted vests

And you don't need to rush off to buy any of these pieces of equipment; there are plenty of creative ways you can make your own resistance training equipment:

- Furniture, such as a chair, table or coffee table and your own body weight
- Objects found out-and-about, such as stairs, park benches, chin-up bars, hills, and your own body weight
- Homemade dumbbells, from any heavy object you can hold, such as wine bottles or tin cans; bottles filled with rocks, sand or water; loaded bags or suitcase; bricks; heavy books such as phone books
- Homemade barbell using a broom or mop handle with ankle weights or bags of rice strapped to either end.

Examples of resistance workouts

- Circuit training
- Climbing a set of stairs
- Lifting weights
- Using machine weights at the gym
- Using a resistance band at home or in the park
- Using your own body weight for exercises like push-ups
- Using your loaded shopping bags for some upper body exercises before you unpack the groceries
- Doing body weight exercises using chairs, tables, steps, chin-up bars and so on
- Pump class (resistance based class using specially made barbells and interchangeable weights)
- Piggybacking a partner and doing squats and carrying them up a hill
- Strapping on ankle weights and doing some lower body exercises
- Doing resistance exercises in the water, with water or aqua dumbbells acting as resistance

- Pushing a pram uphill
- Running/walking up hills
- Running/walking with a weighted vest
- Using a medicine ball for upper body, lower body, and abdominal work

Reasons to join the resistance

Stronger body: Weight bearing exercise strengthens your musculoskeletal system, helping you carry out common activities like carrying groceries and lifting your child. A strong body and bones also assists in preventing falls, and fractures from falling, as we age.

Boosted metabolism: The more muscle you have the more fat you burn. Resistance training is superior in building metabolic muscle.

Burns calories: Lifting weights in a circuit fashion—moving quickly from one exercise to the next, with little or no rest in between—consisting of compound exercises (exercises calling on more than one muscle group, rather than just one muscle group) can actually burn as many calories as going for a run, and offer cardiovascular benefits.

Good posture: A well-balanced body equals good posture; a specifically designed resistance program can rehabilitate injury and strengthen weak muscles, to ensure the body is in balance thus helping to also prevent injury.

Reduced risk of heart disease: It's not just aerobic exercise that has healthy heart benefits. Studies have shown that regular resistance training can also offer cardiovascular benefits and lower blood pressure.

Anti-osteoporosis effect: Weight training is superior in building, and slowing the loss of, bone mineral content, which is essential for reducing the risk of osteoporosis.

Weight loss FAQ

Q: Can you spot reduce?

A: No. You may be able to tone muscles in a specific location but you can't burn fat from a selected location by using the muscles in that area.

Muscle tone: Firm, shapely muscles improve your body shape.

Type 2 diabetes management: Studies show regular strength training helps people with type 2 diabetes to reduce and control their blood glucose levels and improve long-term health complications.

Slows muscle loss: The older we get, and the more crash diets we've been on, the slower our metabolism. This is due to a loss of lean muscle tissue. As we age we lose muscle tissue and strength training counteracts this loss.

Cardio exercise—for stamina

Cardio exercise means any type of rhythmical activity done with the use of oxygen. This is also called 'aerobic' exercise, and is commonly done using large muscle groups—think walking, running, swimming, cycling and so on—for a continuous period of time past around 90 seconds. Just think working the heart and lungs! A cardio workout is usually done at a moderate intensity, so your heart and breathing rate is slightly faster but you could still maintain a conversation with someone while you were exercising—this is commonly referred to as the 'Talk Test' (see 'Measuring Intensity', Chaper 14).

What may be a hard cardio workout for some won't be for others. For example, washing the car may be like doing a cardio session for someone who is unfit but not for a fit person.

Just to confuse matters a little, we have to talk about another type of activity that is commonly done within a cardio workout, called 'anaerobic' exercise. We've just talked about the aerobic system, which is what we mainly use for a cardio session like going for a walk. Here, your heart rate rises and pumps oxygenated blood around your body where it is used for building energy within the muscles in the form of adenosine tri phosphate (ATP). This is the main way our bodies get fuel to function. But say we decided to dash up a steep and long set of stairs whilst on our walk, and the intensity gets too hard? If there's not enough oxygen to meet the increased demands of the new workload, your body switches to another system of energy creation, known as the anaerobic system. Anaerobic simply means working in the absence of oxygen while aerobic exercise means working in the presence of oxygen.

The anaerobic system relies on stored carbohydrates (glucose) in the body over its fat stores, while the aerobic system relies on a combination of carbohydrates and fat.

When you do aerobic exercise, oxygen is used for energy and you're able to keep going for a long time, but when you do anaerobic exercise, your body has enough stored energy to supply the activity only for a short time.

Why are we talking about these technical terms? Well they apply to everyone, not just high-powered athletes. For example, go for a jog and include a few sprints or go for a power walk on a hilly path, and you switch between your aerobic and anaerobic systems. This kind of training has superior benefits for fitness and fat burning, and is what I use for all of my clients, including Chris and Adro's training. You too can learn how to train this way in The Exercise Program (see Chapter 15).

Tools of the trade

- Cardio equipment such as rower, step machine, elliptical trainer, treadmill
- Skipping rope
- Step for step-ups
- Boxing equipment
- Bike

Examples of cardio workouts

- Using cardio equipment
- Running
- Walking
- Cycling
- Swimming

- Rowing

- Dancing

- Boxing/kickboxing

- Skipping

- Aerobic moves on the spot such as star jumps or jogging on the spot

- Aerobics classes

- Hill climbing

- Stair climbing

- Aerobic-based sports, such as soccer and netball

- Dynamic forms of yoga, such as Power Yoga

- Interval training (switching between different exercise intensities)

Reasons to care about cardio

Better body: Cardio, coupled with healthy eating, sheds fat so you can see muscle tone underneath. You could have a six-pack in hiding underneath your belly fat!

Improves cardiovascular fitness: Aerobic exercise conditions your cardiovascular system so you have better heart and lung efficiency.

Stronger heart: Your heart is a muscle and just like any other muscle, it works best when it's conditioned. The more you work it, the fitter it becomes so it doesn't have to work as hard to pump blood around your body.

Lowers your resting heart rate: Regular aerobic exercise can actually lower your resting heart rate. This works in your favour as your heart takes less effort to do the same job.

IF YOU WANT YOUR LIFE TO CHANGE...
YOUR CHOICES MUST CHANGE AND TODAY IS THE BEST DAY OF YOUR LIFE TO BEGIN.

Stress reduction: Effectively manages stress levels, by lowering the stress hormones.

Natural remedy for depression: Large rhythmical forms of aerobic exercise such as swimming, cycling and running have been shown to be most beneficial in dealing with depression.

Disease prevention: Aerobic exercise is a must for conditioning your heart and preventing cardiovascular disease, and reducing the risk of type 2 diabetes, and some cancers.

Better fat burning: Aerobic exercise increases the size and number of mitochondria—the power-stations in your muscle where you burn fat—and is essential for burning enough calories and fat to lose weight.

Improves your cholesterol: Aerobic exercises decrease bad cholesterol (LDL), and increases good cholesterol (HDL).

Improves blood pressure: High BP (hypertension) places excess strain on the heart and can be lowered from long-term exposure to aerobic exercise.

Gives you energy: Pumping oxygen around your body helps to give you energy so you feel less sluggish and more alert for work and life.

Feel good: After a good cardio sweat session, happy hormones are released leaving you on a natural high. More blood and oxygen flow also helps you to look good—people tend to have a natural, healthy glow about them after a good cardio workout.

Boosts your metabolism: Cardio exercise, especially high intensity cardio, raises your metabolism and burns calories post workout.

Stretching—for suppleness

Stretching is often the most neglected part of our training, most people think: 'Well I'm not burning calories or toning muscle when I stretch so who cares'. But stretching is a must for many body benefits, including recovery and injury prevention so you can keep up with your workouts!

Stretching can be static or dynamic. Dynamic stretching means stretching the muscle through movement, while static stretching means taking the muscle to a fully lengthened position and holding—this is the type of stretching most people are familiar with. Stretching is usually done as part of your warm-up and cool-down, but can also be done as a separate session or as part of a yoga class.

Tools of the trade

- Stretching straps
- Resistance bands
- Yoga blocks
- Towel
- Bars
- Fence
- Chair
- Table
- Fitball
- Partner

Stretching Guidelines

The American College of Sports Medicine's stretching guidelines for the general population are: slow, sustained static stretches, three to seven days per week, holding between 10 and 30 seconds. Dont forget to breathe!

Reasons to stretch yourself

Relaxation and stress release: A good stretch relieves muscle tension and tightness, helping your muscles, and you, to relax.

Get more from a workout: Stretching to warm-up helps prepare the body for the movements it has to perform in an upcoming workout. Stretching to cool-down helps relax and restore muscles to their resting length.

Anti-ageing: Stretching can counteract the gradual loss of flexibility that comes with ageing.

Improved flexibility: Tight muscles can lead to many bodily problems—such as headache, aching joints, lower back pain and injury. Stretching or doing yoga improves flexibility and maintains our range of motion (ROM) in our joints, so we feel loose and supple.

Better posture: Prescribed stretches can correct body imbalances occurring from muscle tightness and poor posture—such as a tight chest leading to rounded shoulders or tight hamstrings causing back pain.

More energy and improved circulation: Regular stretching allows oxygen and blood to flow freely through the body.

Reduced risk of injury: We've long been told that we have to stretch to warm-up and reduce our risk of injury … well this isn't entirely true. Researchers have found no solid evidence to suggest that stretching will minimise the risk of injury from participating in sport or exercise. Stretching best helps reduce our risk of injury by helping to keep our body in balance and by removing waste products from our muscles to help muscles recover better.

Physical functioning: A flexible and balanced body improves exercise performance, and even helps with everyday basics such as bending down to shave your legs or to tie a shoe lace.

13. Testing your fitness

Nothing provides greater motivation than results! By monitoring your progress you can get inspired when you see changes. Or, perhaps of even more importance, you can reassess your plan of action if you're not getting the results you're after. There are many ways to evaluate your health and fitness and the ones you do will depend on your goals, but the most common assessments measure the following:

- Blood pressure
- Resting heart rate
- Strength/Strength endurance
- Aerobic fitness
- Flexibility.

Sign up at a gym or with a personal trainer and you will have these aspects of health and fitness assessed. But, there are easy DIY ways to measure your health and fitness that you can do at home. I encourage you to do the tests that follow as a way to see the changes in your health and fitness; this is important because sometimes we may not be losing weight at the rate we like but lose sight of the fact that we are gaining other health and fitness benefits. Keeping a log of the improvements in your health and fitness will show you where your hard work is paying off, even if you're not getting the results you want from the scales, and encourage you to keep going. (Keep a log of these DIY tests in your Weight Loss Journal or in your Testing Diary, see Appendix).

Sports shoe selection

Poor fitting shoes or incorrect footwear (such as wearing a general sneaker for everyday use as well as running and jumping) can cause pain and injury to the lower limbs, such as shin splints, blisters on the feet and knee pain. If the tread on your joggers has worn down or your shoes are so old that they look like your dog's favourite toy, or you're suffering from pain in your feet, ankles, shins or knees during or after exercise then it's probably time to update your sports shoes.

Some buying tips

Shoes must fit well and should not have to be worn in, feeling comfortable straight off.

Shoes must be firm at the front and back of the ankle and your big toe shouldn't be pressing against the front of the shoe.

There are three common foot types: normal foot (ideal), flat foot (pronator) and high arch (supinator); finding a shoe to suit your foot is imperative so you must have it fitted by a professional.

When trying shoes on, wear the same socks you intend to exercise in, try on both feet and walk or run around the shop and try them on in the afternoon as feet have a tendency to swell by this stage of the day.

Once you've bought a pair, to maintain the fit, don't just slip your shoes on and off without undoing the laces and tying them back up again.

Resting heart rate

The resting heart rate (RHR) is the number of times that your heart beats, per minute when totally rested. Exercise results in an increase in the size of the heart. This increase occurs at the cardiac chamber. This means that the heart can eject more blood per beat, and therefore supply the body with the needed blood with less effort.

DIY: Take your pulse

The best time to take your RHR is when you first wake up in the morning.

To take your pulse, sit down and place your first and second fingers on your carotid artery (underneath your chin on the side of your neck) or on the flipside of your wrist. Using a watch or clock to time, measure the number of times you feel it beat in 60 seconds. Most people who are not exercising will usually fall between 70–80 beats per minute (bpm). As your fitness improves your RHR will decrease (the heart is stronger and doesn't have to work as hard).

Ideal heart rate: < 70 bpm.

Cardiovascular endurance

This is one of the most important measures as cardiorespiratory (or heart and lung) fitness gives a true indication of a person's general physical fitness. A person can only exercise as hard as their heart permits so a good score on this test will provide a person with the possibility of faster results, even if they score poorly in some of the other tests. Someone with a low fitness level will have to start out slower than normal and also have shorter work periods during training until they can tolerate the higher loads.

Cardiovascular endurance can be measured in a number of ways—such as charting your heart rate response after walking one kilometre or doing step-ups for a few minutes—most of which are based on the maximal test that directly measures oxygen consumption (VO2max), which simply means the amount of oxygen consumed as you exercise.

DIY: The Timed Run/Walk

This test is used to compare Resting Heart Rates (RHR), Working Heart Rates (WHR), Recovery Heart Rates (Rec HR), and time taken to complete the set distance. As your aerobic fitness improves there will be a reduction in each of these measures. Note: Obtain a health check from your doctor before commencing the test; always warm-up and stretch before commencing; never sit down after finishing—walk around and give your heart rate time to drop down to 120 bpm.

Step 1: Find a course that cannot be altered (so that the distance won't be different when you re-test). For example, the fence at a park or oval, between two houses or fixed points such as telegraph poles. For the best results, the test should be at least 8–15 minutes in duration. This may mean that you must walk the whole way to begin with in order to finish.

Step 2: Measure your RHR before you warm-up.

Step 3: Walk, run or walk/run your course and stop to measure your WHR at regular intervals during the test—such as every kilometre, every two to three minutes, or each time you pass a certain point. Ask a friend to write them down for you.

Step 4: On finishing the course, record the time taken to complete the whole course. For better analysis, record times where you stopped to measure your WHR.

Step 5: Measure your (Rec HR) at the 1st, 2nd, and 3rd minute after finishing. Take this as you're moving about to cool down.

Ideal: Compare your results against your own score when you re-take the test.

Strength/strength endurance

Testing absolute strength is done by seeing the absolute heaviest you can lift once (called a 1RM test), but doing maximum lifts to determine your 1RM is not for beginners. Instead, strength endurance tests are used to see how long your muscles can withstand resistance before fatigue.

DIY: Push-up Test

Complete as many push-ups as possible in 60 seconds. To do a full push-up, place hands and toes on the ground; keep feet together, body straight, and hands under shoulders. Lower down until chest is within 5 centimetres (2 inches) off the floor then push up. Females do the same action but place your knees on the ground (modified push-up). You can see photos for both types of push-up, in Chapter 17.

Ideal:	male	female
Good	>40	>30
Okay	20–39	10–29
Poor	0–19	0–9

DIY: Abdominal Test

Complete as many full crunches in 20 seconds as possible. To do a crunch: lie on the floor with feet on a chair, knees bent at 90 degrees. Fold your arms across your chest with elbows pointing forward. Raise your shoulders off the ground until your elbows touch your thighs. Your elbows must touch the thighs and the shoulders must return to a flat position on the floor for the crunch to be counted. See Chapter 17 for photo of a crunch.

Age	<29	30–39	40–59
Good	>17	>15	>13
Okay	12–17	11–15	10–13
Poor	<12	<11	<10

Flexibility

Flexibility is the ability to move the body's joints through a wide range of motion. The measurement most commonly used in this battery of tests is the Sit-and-Reach Test. This is a widely used test that measures the flexibility of the lower back and hamstrings. Poor flexibility in this area signifies a high chance of lower back injury. Individuals use excuses such as 'my arms are too short', 'my legs are too long', or 'my stomach gets in the way' but none of these factors generally affect flexibility. To be blunt, if you score poorly, then you need to stretch more!

DIY: Sit-and-Reach Test

Sit with your legs straight and feet flat up against a bench or get someone to hold them in position. Reach forward slowly bringing your fingers toward or over your toes as far as you can. Use a tape measure or ruler and measure the gap between your hands and toes (you may need someone to help you with this). Anything before your toes is a negative reading and anything over is positive. Hold for three seconds. Do this three times and take the average. **Ideal:** 1–7cm

14. Exercising for weight loss

Exercise works in two ways when it comes to weight loss: it burns calories and fat, and it raises your metabolic rate post-workout so you keep burning calories for hours after you've taken off your workout gear. But what exercise works best for weight loss? And how do we burn as many calories as we need to in order to lose weight?

Cardio training for weight loss

When exercising for weight loss you need to keep your heart rate above 120 beats per minute (bpm). You can wear a heart rate monitor to get this reading or take your pulse (see Chapter 13) for 15 seconds and multiply by four.

How high should my heart rate go?

Well that depends on your age and fitness level. But, as a general rule of thumb, try to keep it between 120–160 bpm or in a target heart rate zone of 70–85 percent of your maximum heart rate. Some people have their heart rates rise up to 160 bpm just by walking. If this is the case, you don't need to be too concerned, as it will get lower as your fitness improves.

How do I work out my target heart rate zone?

Either go to *www.raykellyfitness.com* to use the calculator, or calculate it yourself by working out the following:

Maximum Heart Rate (MHR) = 220 – age

Heart Rate Reserve (HRR) = MHR – Resting Heart Rate (RHR)

Target Heart Rate (THR) = (HRR x Percentage) + RHR

Below is the calculation for a 30-year-old person, who has a resting heart rate of 70 bpm, to find their target heart rate zone of 70–85 percent MHR:

MHR: 220 – 30 (age) = 190

HRR: 190 – 70 (RHR) = 120

HRR x Percentage: 120 x 0.70 (70 percent for lower training limit) = 84

HRR x Percentage: 120 x 0.85 (85 percent for higher training limit) = 102

Min Heart Rate: 84 + 70 (resting heart rate) = 154

Max Heart Rate: 102 + 70 (resting heart rate) = 172

Therefore, the target heart rate zone for this person would be 154 to 172 bpm.

Will I burn more fat if I exercise in the 'fat-burning zone'?

Fitness professionals were telling people years ago that you should exercise within the 'fat-burning zone', of about 60–75 percent of your maximum heart rate. This is a topic that is truly misunderstood. The body does burn a higher percentage of calories from fat when training at a lower intensity, as well as allowing you to sustain training for longer durations. However, at higher intensities, you burn more total calories during the workout as well as burning calories long after you've finished (helping you to make a greater calorie deficit). High intensity workouts (where you're really huffing and puffing and sweating) have been shown to boost metabolism the most. This is known as the EPOC effect. EPOC stands for Excess Post-exercise Oxygen Consumption. In simple terms, it refers to the energy your body uses after exercise to return itself back to its pre-exercise state. High intensity workouts for longer durations have been shown to boost this effect the most, which will see you burning calories and fat long after your workout.

What's the best cardio for weight loss?

The type of cardio training you choose to do is up to you (see examples in Chapter 12), as long as you can keep your heart rate above 120 bpm. The important thing is to find something that you enjoy and are likely to stick to. No point taking up swimming if you don't enjoy getting wet! Most people find walking best when they are just starting out, then over time they progress to short jogs. Whatever mode of cardio you choose, I recommend that you use a method of training called 'interval training'. I believe that this type of training is superior for fitness and fat loss.

What is interval training?

Put simply, interval training is switching between different levels of intensity, so you alternate between working at a high and low-to-moderate intensity or recovery period. You can do this kind of training using time periods, distance, or just by including intervals at varying intensities. For example, my 15-stage Walk-To-Run Plan in Chapter 15, is based on interval sessions where your hard intervals come

> USE YOUR WORKOUTS AS 'ZONE-OUT' TIME! DON'T BE CONTACTABLE AND DON'T THINK ABOUT WORK.
>
> **Ray Kelly**

from spurts of jogging and your recovery intervals come from bouts of moderate-paced walking. Or, some easy ways to include intervals without thinking about it as much:

- Walk or run on a hilly path

- Walk or run on the beach and alternate between hard and soft sand

- Include a few flights of stairs throughout your walk

- Walk/walk fast or walk/jog every pair of telegraph poles

- Switch between speeds or resistance on cardio equipment

- Intersperse laps of sprinting or deep water running in between your moderate-paced swim

- Alternate between cardio and resistance exercises using a light weight and high reps (repetitions)

- Boxing, punching fast for a time then punching slow for the same time

- When on a bike, stand up for a while then sit down for a while; by standing up you make your body, and butt muscles work harder

- Run, then do a bodyweight exercise, then run again

- Do bouts of sprinting during a run or cycle.

Why is interval training best for weight loss?

Interval training burns more calories than continuous training. When you go on a steady run your heart rate may sit around 150 bpm. But when you're doing intervals, your heart rate may rise to 180 bpm during the intense phase and still maintain 140–150 bpm for the recovery phase. It doesn't end there. Due to the high intensity of the training your body will continue to burn calories for hours afterwards whilst it replaces energy and brings the body's temperature back to normal.

The other benefit of interval training is that it improves your fitness much faster and this in turn enables you to train at higher intensities during all of your cardio work, so even more calories are burned! Several studies have now proved that those who follow a program consisting of interval training lose more weight and get fitter faster than those doing a program of long slow distance

(LSD) training, meaning doing cardio at one slow and steady pace.

Weight training for weight loss

Weight training for weight loss is a lot different to weight-training for muscle building. Building muscle does have its advantages when trying to lose weight but most of us just want to make our muscles firmer and stronger, which is all you need to do to reap the weight loss benefits of weight-training.

How does lifting weights help you lose weight?

The more muscle tissue you have the greater your metabolism because muscle is more metabolically active than fat. So a person of the same size and weight but with more lean muscle tissue than you, is usually burning more calories than you every day. Just by gaining half a kilo (one pound) of muscle you can burn an extra 50 calories a day without doing any extra exercise or activity. Weight training is the best way to build muscle, and this is why it's essential to do some kind of resistance training in a fat loss program.

Weight training also increases muscle strength, which improves your ability to handle anaerobic aspects of your session—such as better leg strength helping you to sprint up a hill or better arm strength to provide you with more power when boxing. Sometimes it's our strength rather than our lungs that limits how fast we can go, so improving this will allow you to work harder during your sessions.

But won't I bulk up?

Some people may feel that they bulk up quite quickly especially if they are shorter in stature, but adding muscle is not that easy. Many men follow muscle building programs for months, doing five to seven workouts a week and eliminating cardio, just to see small increases in muscle size. So you can imagine how hard it is if you're doing loads of cardio, as well as light weights and high reps, which is what the Weight Loss Circuits (see Chapter 16) are based on. And for women it's even harder as you have far less testosterone than men, which contributes to muscle gain.

Program design will contribute greatly to the amount of muscle building that will occur also, so if this is a concern you should avoid doing consecutive exercises on the same muscle group. Muscle building occurs when the individual muscle is continuously fatigued, so you'll have a much less chance of building muscle if you change muscle groups with each exercise (for example, alternate between chest, back, and legs—the Weight Loss Circuits are designed this way). The best way to gauge whether you are actually getting bigger is to take measurements of your waist, hips and stomach, and compare them to past measurements (see Chapter 2).

What's the best weight-training for weight loss?

The best exercises to use for weight loss are compound exercises, rather than isolation exercises, done in a circuit—I call this a compound circuit. Compound exercises use more than one muscle group, so when you're doing the exercise you'll see that more than one joint is moving (for example, when you do a push-up you see your elbow and shoulder joint working); on the other hand, isolation exercises only use one muscle group so you'll notice that only one joint is moving (for example, you only move your elbow joint in a bicep curl).

What's a compound circuit?

Circuit training simply implies moving from one exercise to the next with little or no rest in between. So you're essentially moving from one compound resistance exercise to the next, in a continuous fashion. This differs to the traditional muscle-building program of three sets of 10 repetitions, done in succession with a break in between each set, before moving to the next exercise.

Why is a compound circuit best?

Circuit weight-training allows you to get your heart rate up high without the intense localised fatigue of a muscle-building program. You can lift more weight for each exercise so your strength will increase faster, which will allow you to cope with heavier loads of cardio (calorie and fat burning) exercise.

A program made up of compound exercises burns more calories than one of isolated exercises. Also, compound exercises are usually more functional, which means you strengthen the muscles you use in everyday activities—for example, doing squats strengthens your leg and butt muscles which helps you climb a set of stairs with ease, or bend down to pick up your child, or to get out of a chair. The mechanical stress is shared over all the joints so you have far less chance of injury. This is especially a benefit for those recovering from injury.

The importance of increasing intensity

So you've started a walking program but you're finding it hard to get your heart rate up. This is because your heart is getting stronger. This means it's time to increase the intensity, because you're not burning as many calories, which means you're not burning as much fat, which, you guessed it, means you won't keep losing weight! This is a common mistake many make: they continue doing the same exercise program they began with and wonder why their weight loss slows up.

You need to keep upping the ante to keep getting results. Because your body is such a clever machine, it quickly adapts to a given workload, and becomes so efficient at doing it, that your body almost takes a holiday and does the once-hard session on autopilot. You don't want this to happen. This is why you have to keep 'shocking' the body by giving it new stimulus by increasing the intensity.

When do I have to increase intensity?

Basically, once you feel the workout has become too easy or, despite eating well, your weight loss has stalled—giving your workouts an extra kick along usually gives your weight loss a kick up the backside, too! The rate at which you're ready to increase the intensity depends on your fitness levels. A general guide is five percent per week with an unloading (making no increases) week on the fourth week but if this sounds a little too technical, aim to increase intensity every two weeks or so. Or, in even simpler terms, just let your body be the guide; you will know when you're walking on easy street, and when you need to take it up a gear.

Increase intensity incrementally

Intensity needs to be increased in a step fashion (usually every two to four weeks). Step your workout up a notch, allow some time for things to level out while your body adjusts to the workload, before stepping your workout up again and so on—this is called the training principle of progressive overload. This gives the body time to accommodate to the increased demands you're placing on it, and prevents overloading the body and predisposing yourself to injury.

How do I increase intensity?

You can increase the intensity of your workouts in many different ways, some examples include:

- Changing your walking path to include hills and stairs
- Changing the surface of your walk, runs (sand, grass, road, treadmill)
- Varying the speed or resistance on cardio equipment
- Wearing a weighted vest
- Doing extra repetitions or more sets of a resistance exercise
- Lifting a heavier weight or doing a more challenging exercise
- Introducing new activities/exercises
- Changing from non weight-bearing exercises (rowing, cycling) to weight bearing exercise (cross-trainer, jogging)
- Reduce the rest time between sets when weight-training
- Increasing the work time, or decreasing the recovery time when interval training.

Measuring intensity

You can measure exercise intensity using four common methods:

1. Heart rate: Use a heart rate monitor or take your pulse to make sure your heart rate is above 120 bpm.

2. The Talk Test: If you could talk but not sing and hold a breathy conversation with someone, you're most likely working at a moderate pace; if you can talk but not complete full sentences in between breaths then you're working out at a higher intensity; if you can't utter a word because you're gasping for breath, then you're exercising at your maximum intensity.

3. METs: A general guide on intensity, according to their MET value is:

Low intensity = < 4 METs

Moderate intensity = 4–10 METs

High intensity = > 10 METs

4. Rate of perceived exertion (RPE): The most commonly used RPE guide is the Borg scale, developed by a researcher with the same surname. It rates exercise intensities by numbers and looks like this:

Borg's Rate of Perceived Exertion

6	
7	Very, very light
8	
9	Very light
10	
11	Fairly light
12	
13	Somewhat hard
14	
15	Hard
16	
17	Very hard
18	
19	Very, very hard
20	

Based on this scale, you'd want to be working at around 13–14 for the bulk of your workouts.

> EXERCISE WITH YOUR KIDS! SPEND TIME WITH THE FAMILY AS YOU ALL GET HEALTHY.
>
> **Ray Kelly**

Getting support

Having support for your exercise program can make all the difference in whether or not you stick at it, which for most people is not an easy task; it's usually easy to get motivated to start a workout program, but not so easy to keep at it. Support can come from many sources, such as taking up a team sport (it's much harder to let a whole team down if you don't turn up than it is yourself) joining a cycling club, walking group or mums-with-bubs training group. I recommend you seek support in the following order.

Training partner

Finding a workout buddy can really help you stick to your exercise commitment. They can offer support, guidance, encouragement and a kick up the backside when your workout is slacking off! You want a training partner who is:

Reliable and punctual: They need to be equally committed.

At the same fitness level as you: If they're not you can still train together doing circuit training where you both are free to work at your own individual intensities at each workout station.

Encouraging: Someone who can push you along more than you do yourself.

Supportive and positive: You want someone to uplift you.

Aiming at similar goals: You can then be 'weight loss buddies' and share support and advice on other things such as diet tips, how you beat cravings, your favourite healthy recipes and so on.

Personal trainer

If you prefer to train on your own or get individual encouragement, support, advice and motivation, then a personal trainer is the way to go. If money is an issue you can check in with them fortnightly, or monthly to make sure you're on track and have them teach you new things until you see them next. You want a personal trainer who:

Has experience: An experienced trainer is anyone who has been personal training for over three years.

Has qualifications: Look for one or all of the following: University—Exercise Physiology, Sports Science, Exercise Science, Human Movement, (3 years study); Diploma of Fitness, (6–12 months study); Certificate IV in Fitness, (8 weeks study).

Is insured: Your trainer should have both Public Liability and Professional Indemnity insurance.

Is likeable: Make sure they are someone you can get on with.

Gym

If you can't find a suitable training buddy, workout group or afford personal training, then the gym may be your next bet in finding support. Gyms can be great in offering access to equipment and introducing you to new forms of exercise. You want a gym which provides:

Regularly serviced equipment: Any gym that doesn't service their equipment is not going to service you.

Cleanliness: If a gym is not cleaned daily then the owner is probably cutting costs, which isn't good for a prospective member.

Service: If you don't know much about exercise and nutrition, service is the most important factor of all that you need to look out for. You should be given a new program every 4–6 weeks and another fitness assessment every 8–12 weeks. There should always be someone around to answer your questions.

Your type of clientele: What type of people use the gym at the times you will be training? If you want to avoid bodybuilding types, avoid gyms after 3pm or those gyms which generally have loads of free weights, no aerobic classes, and no (or very old) bikes and treadmills.

Ethics: Are staff constantly trying to push their products? Some unethical centres try to push supplements onto all new members. If the salesperson or instructor seems pushy with their products, run for cover!

Good staff: The most important trait in a good fitness instructor is that they must care. It's easy to identify staff that cares because they are friendly, courteous, and listen!

Reasonable membership price: Every region is different but the membership price should reflect the service, equipment, and instructors. Have a look at a few gyms in your area and compare each one—that is the only reliable way to measure true value.

15. The Exercise Program

Okay, hopefully by now you're feeling exercise-enthused, and can see why it's time to finally make exercise a part of your life if you're serious about losing weight, getting in shape and being in your best health. To help you take up the exercise habit, I want you to follow the following eight steps.

Ray's eight essential exercise steps

Step 1: Visit your doctor

See your doctor for a check-up and medical clearance before you start. Don't worry … it's highly unlikely that they'll say you shouldn't get started. But they will be able to tell you if there are any modifications needed for your exercise program. While you're there, you might like to get some of the tests done that you can't do on your own, such as blood pressure, cholesterol and blood glucose levels. You can keep a record of these in your Testing Diary (see Appendix).

Step 2: Take your tests

Do all of your health and fitness tests (see Chapter 13)—this is important to monitor and measure your progress, as well as document your results. Re-test yourself every 6–8 weeks so you can see how far your fitness has come! Stick at it, and it will improve dramatically in this time frame—you'll see!

Step 3: Increase incidental activity

The first active step in your weight loss plan should be to increase the amount of incidental activity you do—the kind of activity you do outside of planned exercise (check over the ideas listed in Chapter 12). Make a list of ten ways to increase your incidental activity now in your Weight Loss Journal.

Step 4: Plan your exercise

Sit down and plan out your day and you'll see that absolutely everyone can increase the amount of exercise they're getting. The more you exercise, the fitter you get. As we have already discussed the fitter you get, the easier other aspects of your life become—you have more energy, sounder sleep, feel better and have more strength and coordination. Use the Time Management Planner (see Appendix) to work in your planned exercise each day. If you can't find a good 30–60 minute block, then find two shorter workout periods. If you have children you need to find a way to either work it in with them or have someone look after them. If you can't leave the house you can just do laps around the house then complete a body weight circuit. If you still can't find time, you need to increase the amount of incidental activity in your day even further.

Step 5: Get the gear

Okay, so you've scheduled your exercise in for the week, before we plan what exercise you're going to do in these time slots, let's make sure you look the part. The basics for exercise are:

- Cotton t-shirt and/or sweater
- Cotton pants or shorts
- Cotton socks
- Some type of sports shoe (see box on opposite page)
- Lightweight rain jacket (optional)
- Cap or sun-visor if exercising outdoors
- An iPod or MP3 player (optional)—music can motivate you and has been shown to improve exercise performance
- Bike pants (optional)—to prevent chaffing.

Step 6: Choose your exercise program

So you've got the gear sorted, now let's sort out the nitty gritty of your exercise plan. Whatever exercise routine you follow it needs to include resistance and cardio training, and stretching—remember strength, stamina and suppleness (see Chapter 12). To make life easy for you I've mapped out workout plans to factor in each of these training components. Of course, you can design your own training plan or have a personal trainer design a program for you. Whatever you decide, your goal is to come up with an exercise plan that you find enjoyable and facilitates results. This means you will have to allow for flexibility in your programming, and that's why I have given you plenty of variety in the Weight Loss Circuits (see Chapter 16)—there really is something for everyone there! To help you come up with the right exercise plan for you, take a moment to think about your fitness personality. Write your answers in your Weight Loss Journal.

1. Do you enjoy working out in a group or with a training buddy? Or are you more of a lone rider?

2. Where will you feel most comfortable working out? Not fussed? Within convenient distance to home or work? In privacy or small groups? With a personal trainer or at a gym?

3. Make a list of the types of exercise that you enjoy.

4. Now, make a list of the types of exercise that you don't enjoy, but know are good for you!

5. Make a list of any exercise equipment you have lying around the house that you can dust off!

Remember you do not need any exercise equipment to exercise; it's just a bonus that allows you a wider selection of exercise choices. Having a pair of dumbbells is handy for getting the most out of your resistance training. To get started, you can make your own by using any heavy objects around the house. Make a list of what you could use for homemade dumbbells.

Step 7: Mix it up

Once you're into the full swing of your training regime, remember to keep your program fresh by keeping variety in your sessions. A major reason why many people don't stick to their exercise program is boredom.

Try to use at least three different training methods or styles each week, and mix up your exercise choices or even where you exercise. Some suggestions:

- Vary your training methods, switching between walking, running, and boxing for example

- Vary your training styles using continuous, (non-stop activity, e.g., running or walking) intervals (see page 126), sprints, and circuits

- Vary your exercise choices by using different pieces of equipment, your own body weight or dumbbells

- Change the course you take on a regular basis—try the beach, a nature walk, the park, and a walk around your neighbourhood.

Mixing up your sessions also helps to protect against injury from overdoing it with the same exercise, and keeps your body 'awake' as it tries to keep up with the new challenges—this is a must to keep maximising the calories burnt from your exercise program. You'll find that once your fitness improves so, too, will your self-confidence which will inspire you to take on new challenges—perhaps there's something you've always wanted to try, but have been too afraid to or feel that you're too unfit for; set yourself a goal to build enough confidence to give it a try.

Step 8: Keep and review an Activity Diary

Just like your Food Diary, it's important to track your fitness workouts to monitor your results, and assess where things may not be working so well so you can make changes as you need to. It's much easier to have everything down on paper when you're trying to work out why your weight loss isn't progressing. You'll quickly be able to pick up on exercise behaviours—everything from what time of the day you exercise best to what workouts you find yourself regularly skipping! It also makes it easier to do your calorie counting; to make sure you're burning enough from exercise against how much you're putting in from food (which is why you need to keep your Food Diary, too) and also where to make adjustments to burn extra calories through extra exercise if you've had a not-so-good week of eating or you have a special event coming up where you'll be eating extra calories. See the Activity Diary in Appendix.

Now it's time to get down to business and get stuck into your new fitness routine. Simply adapt the exercise plans that follow to suit your lifestyle.

Choosing your exercise plan

Your exercise plan will consist of two components: The Circuits and The 15-stage Walk-to-Run Plan. Within the circuits, there's a range of circuit templates for you to choose from (see Chapter 16, The Weight Loss Circuits) as well as a range of exercises (see Chapter 17, The Exercises). This means you can mix and match and do a different workout every day if you want to!

The Circuits

Aside from the walking and running, the rest of the program consists of Weight Loss Circuits. The circuits are there to: build power, strength and strength endurance; build muscle tissue which boosts metabolism; burn extra calories and offer variety to help maintain interest and exercise adherence.

Which circuit do I do?

There are five types of Weight Loss Circuits to choose from.

Body weight circuit: For those who have no equipment and would like to train anywhere, such as at home.

Compound circuit: If you have free weights, or have access to a home gym or fitness centre, you can try these workouts.

Boxing circuit: Great for variety as in this form of cardio training you're using much more upper body so it gives your lower limbs a rest from walking/running, but also good if you just love boxing.

Cardio circuit: Ideal for those who have access to cardio machines (bike, treadmill, cross-trainer and so on) and enjoy high intensity workouts.

Outdoor circuit: If you like getting fresh air while you're exercising then this style of training is for you.

Simply choose the type of circuit you'd enjoy doing the most, but remember that variety is important so try to mix it up a bit. You can choose which circuits you like based on what equipment you have available and according to your exercise preferences.

Ray's three favourite circuits

1. Outdoor circuit

What is it? Using the resources you have around you—such as hills, gutter steps, sandpits, stairs, park benches—to complete a circuit. You can also take along tools such as dumbbells, or a medicine ball. These are the circuits I predominately did with Adro and Chris. Basically you're running to a station, completing the exercise, then running to the next one. Check out this circuit in Chapter 16.

Why it works. By doing circuit training you get to see an improvement in strength while also increasing cardio fitness, and burning up a stack of calories. By taking your circuit outdoors you'll find it much more interesting than training between four walls, making you less likely to get bored. Sessions can be easily changed each workout, by drawing on the objects around you so you don't have to keep repeating the same session. Try it! You'll work hard without even realising it!

2. Cardio circuit

What is it? We get the heart rate up using a combination of aerobic and anaerobic activity, then jump on a few weight-training exercises (without a break) before getting back on to the intervals again, and repeating the whole process again. Check out this circuit in Chapter 16.

Why it works. In this format, it's easy to use the forms of energy we just talked about: aerobic and anaerobic systems (see page 114). You can train at very high intensities with very low impact.

Intensity can be adjusted and controlled quite accurately by adjusting weights and/or speeds. There is lots of exercise variety available in one small space. All you need is some cardio equipment and a few machines and by changing the variables each day (weight, reps, sets, rest interval, speed, incline and so on) you have a completely new workout.

3. Boxing circuit

What is it? Boxing for exercise isn't about going a few rounds in the ring with a world champion, instead it's more like a 'boxing circuit', borrowing all of the boxing methods and adapting them into an accessible workout for everyone. You can either pair up with someone and box against focus mitts, or you can go solo by setting up a boxing bag at home or a dummy stand—specially designed to withstand a few knocks! Or you can even shadow box—no equipment necessary. Check out this circuit in Chapter 16.

Why it works. Not only is boxing great for fitness and burning loads of calories, it can be done from a standing position, which makes it great for the very overweight and obese where activities like walking and jogging can place undue strain on the joints of the lower body and back. Boxing has the added benefits of improving coordination, fitness, and concentration. It's very easy to adjust a session to your individual fitness level. It's also very easy to change its structure to provide more variety.

Why so much variety?

Variety is very important; it keeps things fresh, provides a constant challenge for your body and prevents you from getting bored so you can enjoy (yes, enjoy!) exercise. Having so much variety also enables you to pick and choose which exercises are best for you, depending on the equipment you have available and what you feel like doing, and to provide constant stimulation so your workout routine never gets stale.

A one-size-fits-all program doesn't suit everyone—we have different needs, different likes and dislikes and different equipment available. So the weight loss circuit templates provide plenty for you to do whether you do or don't have equipment.

How many times do I do a circuit?

Be sure to do the number of circuits per week suggested for each stage (see 'Putting it all together' in this Chapter). For extra fitness and fat-burning (remember that Chris and Adro did multiple sessions a day) you can do more than the specified amount of circuits, but never more than three extra per week. When adding another circuit be sure not to do it back-to-back with any other sessions. It's best to add it in to the opposite end of the day (for example, do one session in the morning, and one in the afternoon).

Can I do these circuits on consecutive days?

Yes! There is no reason why you need to wait 48 hours (the usual recommended rest period in between weight-training sessions) between the resistance-based training circuits when following this format.

Now, the same can't be said for a bodybuilding style program because quite often you're also doing 9–15 sets of the same muscle group back to back. Obviously, doing this type of workout each day would lead to injury.

The Weight Loss Circuits are quite varied. You are never working the same muscle group back to back, you are lifting much lighter weights, and you are sharing the load of each workout across the whole body.

There is nothing wrong with doing two days of circuit then one day off, followed by two more days of circuit.

How many reps and sets do I do in the circuit?

Rep is short for repetition, and refers to how many times you do the exercise, such as 10 push-ups. Sets refers to how many times you complete one set of reps, for example, doing 10 push-ups, having a little rest and then doing another 10 push-ups is doing two sets of 10 reps.

Each exercise has 'Low Reps' and 'High Reps' specified. When someone is just starting they will do the number recommended for the low reps and strive to build up to the high reps. Start with two sets and build up to four sets.

How long do I rest for in between exercise and sets?

Take a little rest to recover, if you need to, and work up to having no rest in between exercises and sets.

How do I warm-up and cool-down?

Walk or do a light jog (or anything that's of low impact and gives you a light sweat) for five minutes before and after your workout followed by stretching. Keep static stretching short at the beginning of the session, say about five stretches, and stretch longer afterwards. Hold stretches for 10–30 seconds.

A warm-up is done at the beginning of a workout, usually for around five minutes and includes light activity (usually a similar activity you're doing for your workout, such as an easy shuffle before going for a run) followed by some static stretching or range-of-motion stretches that mimic the moves you're about to do (such as running drills), and is good for preparing your body for the workout ahead by gradually raising your heart rate and warming your muscles.

A cool-down is done at the end of your workout for around the same time, and includes a bigger stretching component consisting of static stretches, and helps your body (heart rate, breathing and blood pressure) return to normal as well as helping rid waste products from your muscles to help you back up for tomorrow's session with less stiffness.

Here are some useful stretches (see the end of Chapter 17)—do these for your warm-up and cool-down:

- Overhead push
- Chest stretch 1 and 2
- Shoulder stretch
- Standing quadricep stretch
- Seated hamstring stretch
- Standing calf stretch

Add extra stretches to your cool-down for a relaxation and recovery boost.

The 15-stage Walk-to-Run (WTR) Plan

The fastest way to lose weight and increase fitness is to exercise at higher intensities. The problem is though, that most people can't exercise at a high intensity for long. Well, this is where the 15-stage Walk-to-Run (WTR) Plan comes in! The WTR Plan is a progressive cardio plan to build your running fitness and burn calories.

Combine this plan with a weekly amount of circuits that can be chosen from any of the Weight Loss Circuits in Chapter 16.

The workout plans have been modelled on the training I did with Chris and Adro in the seven weeks they had to train with me, outside of *The Biggest Loser* house, in the lead-up to the grand finale where they won! By following this style of training Adro was able to progress from only being able to run for 3 minutes to a full 60 minutes in just five weeks! And my wife used the plan to get her pre-pregnancy body back—she started the program 12 weeks after having our first child, entering at Stage 7, running in 60 second bursts, and within six weeks she was at Stage 14, and running for 45 minutes, not to mention six kilograms lighter! It doesn't matter whether you can only walk for a short period or you're a capable runner, by following the training plan, and eating right, you can expect to lose at least half a kilo a week.

What is it?

This is a progressive 15-stage program that provides you with a full weekly training regime. Simply start at the stage that corresponds with your current fitness level and move forward as your fitness improves.

Who should do it?

People of all fitness levels who want to lose weight and improve their fitness!

Who shouldn't do it?

People who have an injury to their lower body that limits their ability to walk or run. Also, those who have an injury or condition and have been instructed by a professional to not do running, and for whom walking does not raise their heart rate over 120 bpm, should instead replace the walking and running with cardio equipment such as the stepper, cross-trainer, or bike. If you don't have access to this try swimming or cycling.

The 15 stages

Each of the stages require you to do 5–7 workouts consisting of walking/running and a set amount of circuits for the week, which are designed to help you build up to being able to run for continuous periods of time. You can allocate each workout to a day that suits your lifestyle. This style of training works because the workouts are varied and they change as you improve. They also gradually increase in intensity so you are always improving. (See 'Putting it all together' in this chapter).

Moving on to the next stage

Once every two weeks you must test yourself by trying for the next level. Check the prerequisites then test yourself by trying to run for that period of time. You cannot skip levels, and you must spend at least one week on each stage before moving on.

Does the 'no pain, no gain' rule apply?

No. It's important to start your exercise at a steady pace then increase the intensity as your body adapts. This is why the program only allows you to move to the next stage once you have fulfilled the prerequisite for each stage.

At what speed should I run?

You don't have to run fast, even a shuffle is beneficial. As your fitness increases it's important that you push yourself harder, especially for the running intervals.

Why only walking and running?

Walking and running is accessible to everyone, and is fuss-free—no need for cardio equipment, bikes, gyms or pools. But you can easily adjust the program to suit other forms of cardio. Simply adjust the intensities according to Rate of Perceived Exertion (RPE) scale (see Chapter 14). Consider what pace would provide you with a good workout when you're going at the same pace throughout the workout (most likely a RPE of 13). This means your high intensity intervals (where it says jog) should be a RPE of around 15, and the recovery intervals a RPE of around 11.

Keep it interesting

Change the course of your walks/runs regularly to maintain variety and keep you stimulated. To also help prevent injury, vary your training surfaces: try the road, grass on an oval, footpath, running track, bushwalk track, treadmill and sand (when you're ready for an extra challenge!).

Why so often?

Workouts are scheduled for 5–7 days a week. The single biggest factor for succeeding with an exercise program is consistency. What you do is nowhere near as important as how often you do it. Yes, exercising three times per week will improve your health but it won't change your lifestyle. We need to get you to start being active every day. That is how you get results!

Also, planning to exercise each day of the week helps you to stay focused, by not giving you an 'out'. If you plan three sessions a week, you've got four days to allow for the 'I'll do it tomorrow' excuse, which rarely happens! By accepting that you need to exercise every day it's likely to become a habit—not to mention make you less likely to succumb to food temptations ('I've been good with exercise, I don't want to ruin it by eating incorrectly').

Exercise intensity

Remember that it's best to exercise between 70 percent and 85 percent of your maximum heart rate. For most people this will be between 120 and 160 beats per minute (bpm), and beginners will usually reach this just by walking. Everyone's heart rate is different, and is based on such factors as age, fitness level, health conditions, and medications taken. If you think that this range is unrealistic for you or it causes you any concern please discuss it with your doctor. For ways to measure exercise intensity, see Chapter14.

Putting it all together

It's time to put those walking shoes on, choose the circuits that appeal to you and get started! Remember:

- Do a little cardio session to see where you're up to

- Start at the stage that you can complete the prerequisites

- Re-test every two weeks and adjust

- Remember to warm-up and cool-down

For example, Stage 5 looks like this: On one day, walk fast for 30 minutes. On another day, run for 10 seconds, walk for 5 minutes and complete 6 times. On another, run for 10 seconds, walk for 3 minutes and complete 10 times. On two days in that week, walk for an hour each day. On another two, choose two circuits from Chapter 16 such as Body Weight Circuit 1 and Boxing Circuit 2 and complete one on each of those days. It doesn't matter which day each session is done on as long as they're all done in the week.

Stage 1: Walk for 5 minutes

Prerequisite: Must be able to walk 5 minutes non-stop

Weekly Program: Walk for 5 minutes each day on a flat surface

Stage 2: Walk for 10 minutes

Prerequisite: Must be able to walk 10 minutes non-stop

Weekly Program: Walk for 10 minutes daily, using at least three courses throughout the week

Starter circuit x 3: 10 reps of Squats, Wall Push-Ups, and Crunches: 3 sets of each

Stage 3: Walk for 20 minutes

Prerequisite: Must be able to walk 20 minutes non-stop

Weekly Program:

5 x 20 minute walks per week. Two of these should be on a 'hilly' course (not mountainous though!)

2 x circuits

Stage 4: Walk for 40 minutes

Prerequisite: Must be able to walk 40 minutes non-stop

Weekly Program:

2 x 20 minute walks per week at a faster pace than your 40 minute walks

3 x 40 minute walks per week. At least one of these should be on a 'hilly' course

2 x circuits

Stage 5: Walk for 60 minutes

Prerequisite: Must be able to walk 60 minutes non-stop, and jog for 10 seconds

Weekly Program:

1 x 30 minute walk at a fast pace

1 x interval session: 10 second run, 5 minute walk x 6

1 x interval session: 10 second run, 3 minute walk x 10

2 x 60 minute walks

2 x circuits

Stage 6: Jog for 30 seconds

Prerequisite: Must be able to jog for 30 seconds non-stop, and walk 60 minutes non-stop

Weekly Program:

2 x 60 minute walk

1 x interval session: 30 second run, 5 minute walk x 7

1 x interval session: 30 second run, 3 minute walk x 5

1 x interval session: 15 second run, 1 minute walk x 8

2 x circuits

Stage 7: Jog for 60 seconds

Prerequisite: Must be able to jog for 60 seconds non-stop, and walk 60 minutes non-stop

Weekly Program:

1 x 60 minute walk

1 x interval session: 60 second run, 5 minute walk x 6

1 x interval session: 60 second run, 3 minute walk x 4

1 x interval session: 30 second run, 2 minute walk x 6

1 x interval session: 15 second run, 1 minute walk x 10

2 x circuits

Stage 8: Jog for 2 minutes

Prerequisite: Must be able to jog for 2 minutes non-stop, and walk 60 minutes non-stop

Weekly Program:

1 x 60 minute walk

1 x interval session: 2 minute run, 8 minute walk x 3

1 x interval session: 2 minute run, 6 minute walk x 4

1 x interval session: 60 second run, 3 minute walk x 6

1 x interval session: 30 second run, 2 minute walk x 10

2 x circuits

Stage 9: Jog for 5 minutes

Prerequisite: Must be able to jog for 5 minutes non-stop, and walk 60 minutes non-stop

Weekly Program: 1 x 60 minute walk

1 x interval session: 5 minute run, 20 minute walk x 2

1 x interval session: 5 minute run, 10 minute walk x 3

1 x interval session: 2 minute run, 6 minute walk x 5

1 x interval session: 60 second run, 3 minute walk x 10

2 x circuits

Stage 10: Jog for 10 minutes

Prerequisite: Must be able to jog for 10 minutes non-stop, and walk 60 minutes non-stop

Weekly Program:

1 x 60 minute walk

1 x continuous session: 10 minute run, 30 minute walk

1 x interval session: 10 minute run, 10 minute walk x 2

1 x interval session: 5 minute run, 10 minute walk x 3

1 x interval session: 2 minute run, 6 minute walk x 5

2 x circuits

Stage 11: Jog for 15 minutes

Prerequisite: Must be able to jog for 15 minutes non-stop

Weekly Program:

1 x 60 minute walk

2 x continuous sessions: 15 minute run, 30 minute walk

1 x interval session: 10 minute run, 15 minute walk x 2

1 x interval session: 5 minute run, 10 minute walk x 3

2 x circuits

Stage 12: Jog for 20 minutes

Prerequisite: Must be able to jog for 20 minutes non-stop

Weekly Program:

1 x 60 minute walk

2 x continuous sessions: 20 minute run, 20 minute walk

1 x interval session: 10 minute run, 10 minute walk x 2

1 x interval session: 5 minute run, 10 minute walk x 4

2 x circuits

Stage 13: Jog for 30 minutes

Prerequisite: Must be able to jog for 30 minutes non-stop

Weekly Program:

1 x 60 minute walk

2 x continuous sessions: 30 minute run

1 x interval session: 10 minute run, 10 minute walk x 3

1 x interval session: 5 minute run, 5 minute walk x 5

2 x circuits

Stage 14: Jog for 45 minutes

Prerequisite: Must be able to jog for 45 minutes non-stop

Weekly Program:

1 x 60 minute walk

2 x continuous sessions: 45 minute run

1 x continuous session: 30 minute run

1 x interval session: 10 minute run, 5 minute walk x 4

1 x interval session: 2 minute run, 2 minute walk x 10

1 x circuit

Stage 15: Jog for 60 minutes

Prerequisite: Must be able to jog for 60 minutes non-stop

Weekly Program:

1 x 60 minute walk

2 x continuous sessions: 60 minute run

1 x continuous session: 40 minute run

1 x interval session: 15 minute run, 5 minute walk x 2

1 x interval session: 1 minute run, 1 minute walk x 10

1 x circuit

16. The Weight Loss Circuits

Whether you're using a home-gym, machine weights at the gym, free-weights at home or no equipment at all will determine which exercises you can do, as well as which exercises you enjoy. I've provided the following circuits for you. See Chapter 17 for all the exercises

Body weight circuit: No equipment required; on each line write in one exercise you choose from the Body Weight exercises, and do the same for the Abdominal exercises, the Plyometrics exercises and the Rhythmic exercises.

Compound circuit: Weights required; on each line write in one exercise you choose from the Compound circuit exercises which work that particular muscle group listed. On the lines next to the 'Abdominals', write in one exercise you choose from the Abdominal exercises.

Boxing circuit: No equipment required; on each line write in one exercise you choose from the Boxing exercises, and do the same for the Plyometrics exercises.

Cardio circuit: Cardio equipment required; on each line write in one exercise you choose from the Body Weight exercises, and do the same for the Abdominal exercises, and the Plyometrics exercises.

Outdoor circuit: Cones or suitable markers, such as items of clothing, shoes or drink bottles required; on each line write in one exercise you choose from The Exercises (Chapter 17) or do the specified exercises.

When starting out just complete each circuit through twice and build up to 3–4 times. If you need a break between each exercise in the beginning that's fine but try to build up to no break. If you can't skip or have no rope just pretend you have a rope. Only skip for 30–60 seconds. Warm-up and cool-downs must be added.

Body weight circuit

Body Weight Circuit 1

Body Weight _____

Abdominals _____

Body Weight _____

Abdominals _____

Body Weight _____

Abdominals_____

Body Weight_____

Abdominals _____

Body Weight Circuit 2

Body Weight _____

Skipping _____

Abdominals _____

Body Weight _____

Skipping _____

Abdominals _____

Body Weight _____

Skipping _____

Abdominals _____

Body Weight Circuit 3

Body Weight _____

Plyometrics _____

Abdominals _____

Body Weight _____

Plyometrics _____

Abdominals _____

Body Weight _____

Plyometrics _____

Abdominals _____

Body Weight Circuit 4

Body Weight _____

Rythmic _____

Abdominals _____

Body Weight _____

Rythmic _____

Abdominals _____

Body Weight _____

Rythmic _____

Abdominals _____

Compound Circuits

Compound Circuit 1

Chest _____

Legs _____

Back _____

Abdominals _____

Chest _____

Legs _____

Back _____

Abdominals _____

Chest _____

Legs _____

Back _____

Compound Circuit 2

Chest _____

Legs _____

Abdominals _____

Back _____

Chest _____

Abdominals _____

Legs _____

Back _____

Abdominals _____

Compound Circuit 3

Chest _____

Abdominals _____

Back _____

Abdominals _____

Legs _____

Abdominals _____

Chest _____

Abdominals _____

Back _____

Abdominals _____

Legs _____

Abdominals _____

Boxing Circuit

Box for 60 seconds and build up to 2 minutes over the course of a few months. If you can't skip or have no rope just pretend you have a rope. Only skip for 60 seconds.

Boxing Circuit 1

Boxing _____

Skipping _____

Boxing _____

Skipping _____

Boxing _____

Skipping _____

Boxing _____

Skipping _____

Boxing _____

Skipping _____

Boxing _____

Skipping _____

Boxing _____

Skipping _____

Boxing _____

Skipping _____

Boxing Circuit 2

Boxing _____

Plyometrics _____

Skipping _____

Boxing _____

Plyometrics _____

Skipping _____

Boxing _____

Plyometrics _____

Skipping _____

Boxing _____

Plyometrics _____

Skipping _____

Boxing _____

Plyometrics _____

Skipping _____

Boxing _____

Plyometrics _____

Skipping _____

Boxing _____

Plyometrics _____

Skipping _____

Boxing _____

Plyometrics _____

Skipping _____

Boxing Circuit 3

Boxing _____

Skipping _____

Abdominals _____

Boxing _____

Skipping _____

Abdominals _____

Boxing _____

Skipping _____

Abdominals _____

Boxing _____

Skipping _____

Abdominals _____

Boxing _____

Skipping _____

Abdominals _____

Boxing _____

Skipping _____

Abdominals _____

Boxing _____

Skipping _____

Abdominals _____

Boxing _____

Skipping _____

Abdominals _____

Cardio circuits

These circuits are for those who have one or more pieces of cardio equipment. If you are using a treadmill, a hard pace will be a few kilometres per hour over what you'd normally do for five minutes. If that means running and you are unable to run, increase the incline. If you are using a bike you have two options: Stand up for the hard periods (you'll have to increase the intensity so the pedalling remains smooth) and sit down for the light. Otherwise, stay seated for both hard and light but increase the intensity for the hard period.

If you are using a rowing machine, decrease the split time per 500 metres (the number in the large box in the middle) for the hard period, and decrease for the light.

If you are using a cross-trainer, the hard period should be a few levels above what you'd normally do for five minutes. The light period will be a few levels below what you'd normally do for five minutes.

Cardio circuit 1

Body Weight _____

Plyometrics _____

Abdominals _____

Cardio (30s hard, 30s light, x 2) _____

Body Weight _____

Plyometrics _____

Abdominals _____

Cardio (30s hard, 30s light, x 2) _____

Body Weight _____

Plyometrics _____

Abdominals _____

Cardio (30s hard, 30s light, x 2) _____

Cardio circuit 2

Body Weight _____

Skipping _____

Abdominals _____

Cardio (2min hard, 2min light) _____

Body Weight _____

Skipping _____

Abdominals _____

Cardio (2min hard, 2min light) _____

Body Weight _____

Skipping _____

Abdominals _____

Cardio (2min hard, 2min light) _____

Cardio circuit 3

Body Weight _____

Abdominals _____

Body Weight _____

Cardio (20s hard, 40s light, x 3)_____

Body Weight _____

Abdominals _____

Body Weight _____

Cardio (20s hard, 40s light, x 3) _____

Body Weight _____

Abdominals _____

Body Weight _____

Cardio (20s hard, 40s light, x 3) _____

Cardio circuit 4

Chest _____

Legs _____

Cardio (30s hard, 60s light, x 2)_____

Back _____

Abdominals _____

Cardio (30s hard, 60s light, x 2) _____

Chest _____

Legs _____

Cardio (30s hard, 60s light, x 2) _____

Back _____

Abdominals _____

Cardio (30s hard, 60s light, x 2)_____

Outdoor circuit

Outdoor Circuit 1

- Place cones 20–50 metres apart depending on fitness level. Select 5 exercises from the plyometric section, and 5 from the body weight section.

- Start at cone 1 and run to cone 2, complete 10 sit-ups then continue to cone 3 (where you will do one of the body weight exercises).

- Run back to cone 2, do 5 push-ups then run to cone 1 (where you will do one of the plyometric exercises).

- Continue until all exercises are done.

- Complete 2–3 times, with 5 minutes break between each full circuit.

Modifications: Running forward can be changed to sideways or backwards for variety. Running can be exchanged for walking to decrease intensity.

Outdoor Circuit 2

- Place cones 10 metres apart. Select 2 exercises from the body weight section, 2 from the plyometric section, and 1 from the abdominal section.

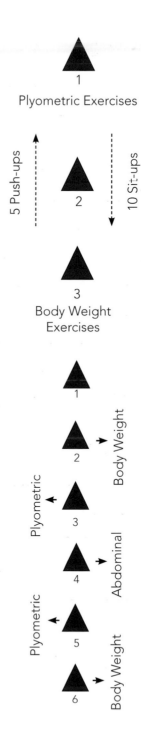

- Starting at cone 1, run to cone 2 and complete the exercise for that station, then run back to cone 1.

- Repeat for cones 3, 4, 5, and 6. Complete 3 times.

- Complete 2–3 times, with 5 minutes break between each full circuit.

Modifications: Running forward can be changed to sideways or backwards for variety. Running can be exchanged for walking to decrease intensity.

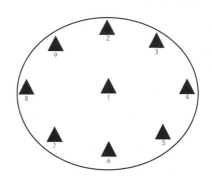

Outdoor Circuit 3

- Set up 1 cone in the middle of an oval/football field, and 8 cones around the perimetre.

- Starting at cone 1, run to cone 2 and complete a plyometric exercise, then run back to cone 1.

- Repeat for cones 3, 4, 5, 6, 7, 8, and 9. Complete 3 times, doing a different exercise at each cone.

- Complete 2–3 times, with 3 minutes break between each full circuit.

Modifications: Running forward can be changed to sideways or backwards for variety. Running can be exchanged for walking to decrease intensity.

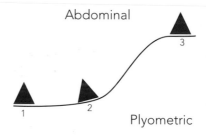

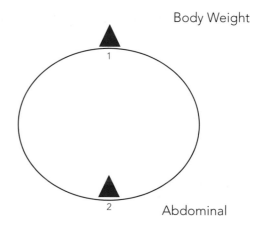

Outdoor Circuit 4

- Set up a cone at your starting position (1), the foot of a small hill/incline (2), and at the top of the hill/incline (3). Select 5 exercises from the plyometric section, and 5 from the abdominal section.

- Run to cone 2, complete the first plyometric exercise, then run to cone 3 and complete the first abdominal exercise. Run back to cone 1. Repeat until all exercises are done.

- Complete 2–3 times, with 3 minutes rest between each full circuit.

Modifications: Running forward can be changed to sideways or backwards for variety (except downhill). Running can be exchanged for walking to decrease intensity

Outdoor Circuit 5

- Set cones up at halfway points on an oval/ football field. Select 8 exercises from the body weight section, and 8 from the abdominal section.

- Starting at cone 1, run to cone 2 and complete the first exercise on that list. From there, run to cone 1 and complete the first on that list.

- Continue through until you've done all exercises.

Modifications: Running can be exchanged for walking to decrease intensity

17. The Exercises

Use the following exercises to complete the Weight Loss Circuits in the previous chapter to incorporate in your exercise program. You can follow the circuits I've outlined for you, then when you're more confident all you have to do is mix and match according to what exercise equipment you have and what exercises you like to do, using the templates. The circuits include a selection of the following:

- Compound circuit exercises
- Abdominal exercises
- Lower back exercises
- Body weight exercises
- Plyometric exercises
- Rhythmic exercises
- Boxing exercises
- Stretches—for warm-up and cool-down.

1st Beginner: This exercise is suitable for someone just starting out

Back: If you have a history of back injury, take caution with this exercise

Knee: If you have a history of knee injury, take caution with this exercise

Ankle: If you have a history of ankle injury, take caution with this exercise

Shoulder: If you have a history of shoulder injury, take caution with this exercise

Blood Pressure: If you have high blood pressure, take caution with this exercise

Compound circuit exercises

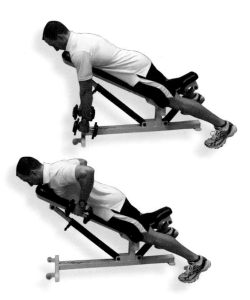

Bench Row (1st)

Muscle Group: Back

Set incline bench to allow for full extension of the arms. Lie face down on bench, feet touching floor with knees slightly bent. With your arms fully extended, pull dumbbells up towards your chest keeping elbows high. Lower dumbbells to start position.

Tip: Keep chin and chest touching the bench.

Grade: 1   **Low Reps:** 10   **High Reps:** 30

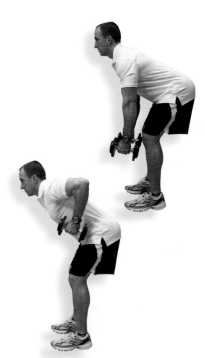

Bent Over Row (Dumbbell)

Muscle Group: Back

Feet shoulder-width apart and knees slightly bent. Lean torso forward, 10–30 degrees above horizontal. Hold a flat-back position, tilt head and look straight ahead. Pull dumbbells up and touch the side of the ribs. Lower dumbbells slowly until arms are fully extended.

Tip: To take pressure off the lower back, rest your head on a bench or bar.

Grade: 2   **Low Reps:** 10   **High Reps:** 30

One Arm Row

Muscle Group: Back

Place inside hand and knee on bench. Position torso parallel with floor, keeping knee under hip and hand under shoulder. Hold dumbbell with outside hand. Hang dumbbell with arm straight. Raise dumbbell up toward the hip, keeping elbow high. Keep hips and shoulders even and parallel to floor. Touch hip and slowly lower to starting position.

Tip: Ensure that the shoulders stay parallel to the floor throughout the movement. Any rotation means that you are using your lower back and this kind of twisting can lead to injury.

Grade: 1 **Low Reps:** 10 **High Reps:** 30

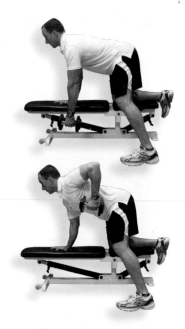

Lat Pulldown

Muscle Group: Back

Hold bar with a closed, pronated, shoulder-width grip. Pull bar down so you are facing the machine with thighs under the pads. Keep torso upright and start with arms fully extended. Pull bar down to top of chest, maintaining body position. Slowly raise bar to starting position.

Tip: To obtain a full contraction, squeeze the elbows towards the ribs. You won't be able to lift as much weight, but you will definitely feel it.

Grade: 1 **Low Reps:** 10 **High Reps:** 30

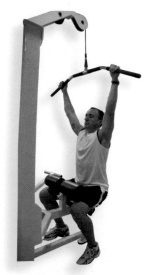

Seated Row 1st

Muscle Group: Back

Sit with torso at 90 degrees to the floor, knees slightly bent. Pull bar towards upper abdomen. Keep body stationary only moving at the elbows and shoulder joints. Touch bar on abs and slowly return to starting position.

Tip: Keep legs slightly bent and lower back stationary. Any rocking forward during this movement may lead to lower back injury.

Grade: 1 **Low Reps:** 10 **High Reps:** 30

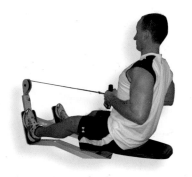

Bench Press, Flat (Barbell) 1st

Muscle Group: Chest

Beginners position feet flat on bench, advanced lifters position feet on floor. Eyes should be below bar. Grasp bar with pronated, slightly wider than shoulder-width grip. Move bar off rack. Position bar over shoulders, arms fully extended. Lower bar slowly and under control, keeping wrists straight. Pause when bar lightly touches chest near the nipples. Push bar up to full elbows extension. Do not arch lower back.

Tip: To check if you are using the correct width grip, lower the bar to the chest. If the forearms are perpendicular to the floor, then you are using the most efficient grip.

Grade: 1 **Low Reps:** 10 **High Reps:** 30

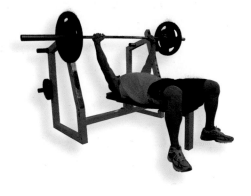

Bench Press, Flat (Dumbbell)

Muscle Group: Chest

Beginners position feet flat on bench, advanced lifters position feet on floor. Position dumbbells over shoulders, arms fully extended. Lower dumbbells slowly and under control, keeping wrists straight. Pause when dumbbells are in line with the top of your chest. Push dumbbells up to full elbow extension. Do not arch lower back.

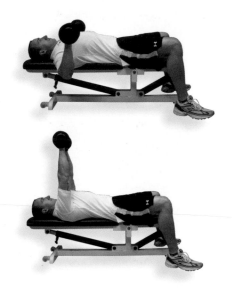

Tip: Ensure that forearms stay perpendicular to the floor throughout the movement. If the dumbbells come in toward the body, the workload of the triceps will increase. This will cause them to fatigue, which will limit the effectiveness of the exercise to train the chest.

Grade: 1 **Low Reps:** 10 **High Reps:** 30

Bench Press, Incline (Dumbbell)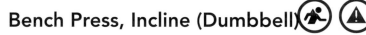

Muscle Group: Chest

Sit on the incline bench, with feet flat on the floor. Keep head, shoulders and butt flat on bench. Press both dumbbells to extended arm position above head. Keeping forearms parallel, lower dumbbells slowly to chest height. Maintain body position on bench, feet on floor. Keeping forearms parallel, press dumbbells to full elbow extension.

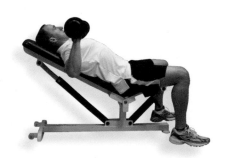

Tip: Keep the bench below 45 degrees. This will limit the amount the shoulders are used and maximise the use of the upper chest!

Grade: 1 **Low Reps:** 10 **High Reps:** 30

High Step (Dumbbell)

Muscle Group: Legs

Box or step should be 30–45 cm high (depending on which height creates a 90 degree angle at the knee joint when foot is on the box). Hold dumbbells so palms are facing inward. Keep shoulders back and torso erect. Step up keeping the knee in line with the toes. Step down and repeat with same leg.

Tip: When stepping up, place your feet so that they run along parallel lines. This will ensure that you are well balanced and will help to work the overall thigh area! Do not lean forward. This causes stress to the lower back and should be avoided.

Grade: 3 **Low Reps:** 10 **High Reps:** 30

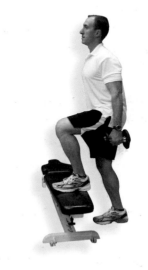

Leg Press (45 degree)

Muscle Group: Legs

Place feet hip-width apart on foot platform. Position thighs, lower legs, and feet parallel to each other. Keep butt on thigh pad and back flat against back pad. Push foot platform forward off rack. Turn rack handles out. Straighten legs (knees still slightly bent). Slowly and under control lower the platform, keeping feet flat. Lower so that a 90 degree angle is achieved at the knee joint. When angle is achieved, push forward on foot platform. Keep thighs, lower legs, and feet parallel to each other. Avoid forcefully locking out knees.

Tip: Lowering the weight below 90 degrees at the knee joint places the knee under considerable stress and should be avoided.

Grade: 1 **Low Reps:** 10 **High Reps:** 30

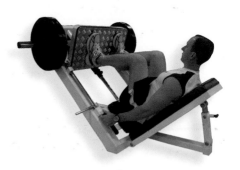

Lunge (Dumbbell)

Muscle Group: Legs

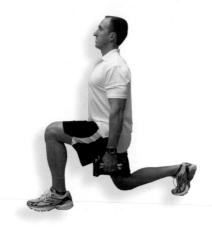

Hold dumbbells so that palms are facing inward. Position feet hip-width apart. Keep head up and torso erect. Take a long step forward with one leg. Do not step to the centre, keep feet along parallel lines. Keep front knee and foot aligned, toes pointing straight ahead. Bend at front knee and slowly lower under control.

Tip: When stepping out in front, place your feet so that they run along parallel lines. This will ensure that you are well balanced and will help to work the overall thigh area.

Grade: 1   **Low Reps:** 10   **High Reps:** 30

Squat (Dumbbell) 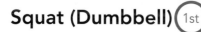 1st

Muscle Group: Legs

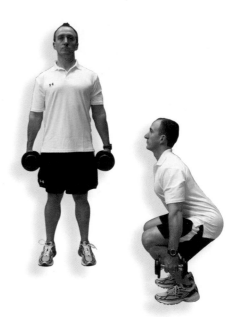

Position feet shoulder-width apart for males, or hip-width apart for females. Keep back straight and pull shoulders back. Focus eyes on wall 30–60 cm above eye level. Slowly and under control, lower dumbbells by bending at the hips and knees. Maintain erect body position. Keep weight over the middle of the feet and heels, and not the toes. Keep heels on the floor. Keep knees aligned with direction of toes. Slowly lower hips until tops of thighs are parallel to floor. After slight pause, slowly return to starting position by straightening hips and knees.

Tip: Make sure that the hips and knees move at the same time. If your hips move before your knees it means that your lower back is getting worked excessively and an injury may occur. You should reduce the weight you are lifting and check your technique.

Grade: 1   **Low Reps:** 10   **High Reps:** 30

Squat (Front)

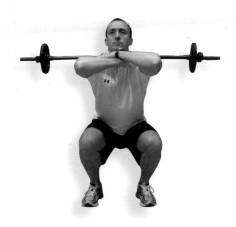

Muscle Group: Legs

Step under the bar and position it evenly across the front of the shoulders. Cross arms and place hands over the bar, and thumbs under bar between the shoulders and neck. Pull shoulder blades toward each other and keep your elbows high. Position feet shoulder-width apart for males, or hip-width apart for females. Focus eyes on wall 30–60 cm above eye level. Slowly and under control, lower bar by bending at the hips and knees. Maintain erect body position. Keep weight over the middle of the foot and heels, not the toes. Keep heels on the floor. Keep knees aligned with direction of toes. Slowly lower hips until tops of thighs are parallel to floor. After slight pause, slowly raise bar by straightening hips and knees.

Tip: Keep bar close to your throat and your elbows high. This will keep your back straight, and free from injury.

Grade: 3   **Low Reps:** 10   **High Reps**: 30

Sumo Squats

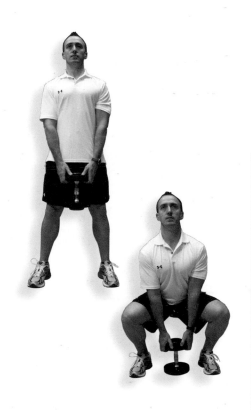

Muscle Group: Legs

Stand with feet slightly wider than hip width. Keeping back straight, hold dumbbell with both hands. Slowly lower dumbbell, keeping back straight. Pause, then use legs to lift back to start position.

Tip: Ensure back is straight throughout the movement.

Grade: 1   **Low Reps:** 10   **High Reps:** 30

High Step Laterals

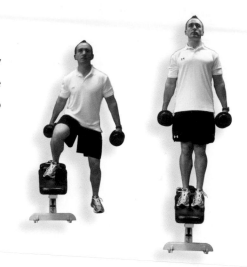

Muscle Group: Legs

Using a chair between 20–30 cm high, step up laterally (sideways). When you step up onto the bench or chair, be sure to place your whole foot down so that you don't slip or trip over.

Tip: Be sure to place your whole foot on the bench.

Grade: 3 **Low Reps:** 10 **High Reps:** 30

Abdominal exercises

Ankle Touches—Legs Up

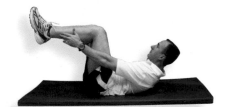

Lying down with your legs up and hands behind head (elbows out of sight). Use your abdominals to lift your shoulder blades off the ground as you extend your left hand towards your left foot. Slowly return to starting position.

Grade: 2 **Low Reps:** 10 **High Reps:** 50

Cross Overs—Knees Up

Lying down with your legs up and hands behind head (elbows out of sight). Use your abdominals to lift your shoulder blades off the ground as you extend your right hand towards your left foot. Slowly return to starting position.

Grade: 2 **Low Reps:** 10 **High Reps :** 50

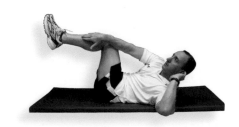

Crunches—Knees Up

Bend your knees at 90 degrees so that your lower legs are parallel to the ground. Use your abdominals to lift your shoulder blades off the ground. Slowly return to starting position.

Tip: To increase the intensity of the abdominal crunch, place hands at side of head (elbows should stay out of sight throughout this movement!).

Grade: 2   **Low Reps:** 10   **High Reps:** 50

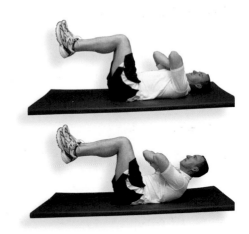

Hip Raises

Lay on your back with your feet flat. Lift bottom off the floor so that your body is straight between the knees and the shoulders.

Grade: 1   **Low Reps:** 10   **High Reps:** 50

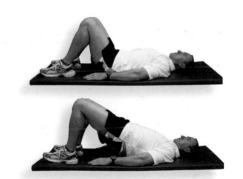

Isometric Knee Push (1st) ⚠

Lay on back, lift feet up and bend knees at 90 degrees. Push lower back into the floor and push on the knees. Hold for 10–60 seconds.

Tip: Do not hold your breath during this exercise as it can cause an increase in blood pressure.

Grade: 1   **Low Reps:** 10 seconds   **High Reps:** 60 seconds

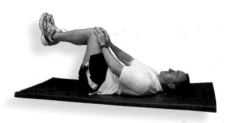

Oblique Isometrics

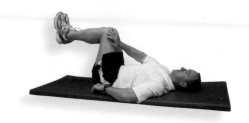

Lay on floor with legs up and bent at 90 degrees. Push lower back into floor. Place right hand on left knee and push. Hold for 10–60 seconds. Repeat for other side.

Tip: Do not hold your breath during this exercise as it can cause an increase in blood pressure.

Grade: 1 **Low Reps:** 10 seconds **High Reps:** 60 seconds

Planks

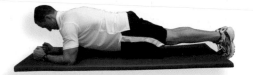

Stay on toes. Keep feet together. Have elbows under the shoulders. Keep body flat. Squeeze your abdominal muscles.

Tip: Do not hold your breath during this exercise as it can cause an increase in blood pressure.

Grade: 1 **Low Reps:** 10 seconds **High Reps:** 60 seconds

Reverse Crunches

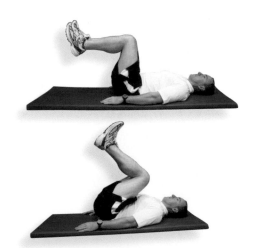

Lift your legs off the floor and bend them at 90 degrees. Use your abdominals to lift your bottom off the floor, squeezing your pelvis towards your chest. Slowly lower to starting position.

Grade: 2 **Low Reps:** 10 **High Reps:** 30

Side Crunches

Lay on your side with knees bent at 90 degrees, hands behind head with elbows pointing towards the sky. Use your obliques to lift your shoulder off the ground, squeezing your elbows towards your hip. Slowly lower to starting position.

Grade: 1   **Low Reps:** 10   **High Reps:** 50

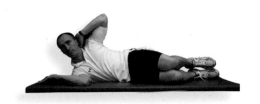

Sit-Ups (Arms crossed   /hands on thighs)

Both feet flat on the ground. Bend knees to 90 degrees. Cross arms on your chest. Use your abdominals to lift your upper body until your shoulder blades are off the ground. Slowly lower to starting position. Beginners can run their hands along their thighs.

Grade: 1   **Low Reps:** 10   **High Reps:** 50

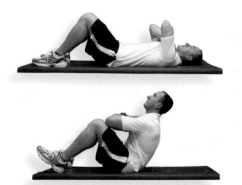

Planks—Knee

Place knees on floor and elbows under your shoulders. Keep body flat. Squeeze your abdominal muscles.

Tip: Do not hold your breath during this exercise as it can cause an increase in blood pressure.

Grade: 1   **Low Reps:** 20 seconds   **High Reps:** 90 seconds

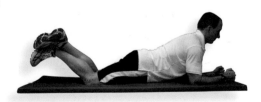

Plank—Arm Raised

Stay on toes. Keep feet together. Have right elbow under the shoulder, with left arm out straight. Keep body flat. Squeeze your abdominal muscles.

Tip: Do not hold your breath during this exercise as it can cause an increase in blood pressure.

Grade: 3   **Low Reps:** 10 seconds   **High Reps:** 60 seconds

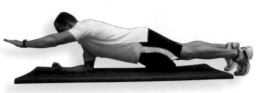

Plank—Side

Keep body straight and shoulders square. Squeeze abdominals.

Tip: Do not hold your breath during this exercise as it can cause an increase in blood pressure.

Grade: 2   **Low Reps:** 10 seconds   **High Reps:** 60 seconds

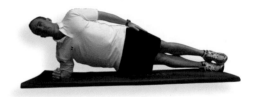

Double Crunches

With feet and hands off the floor, use your abdominals to pull your knees towards your chest while simultaneously lifting your head and shoulders off the ground. Slowly return to starting position.

Grade: 3   **Low Reps:** 5   **High Reps:** 20

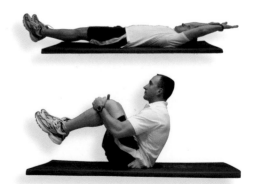

Twisting Iso Crunch

Hold upper body and legs off the floor, balancing on butt. Slowly rotate the upper body to the left, then back to the right. Be sure to rotate at the waist and not just the arms.

Tip: Turn shoulders throughout movement and don't rest elbows on the floor. Use a weight for added resistance.

Grade: 3 **Low Reps:** 10 **High Reps:** 30

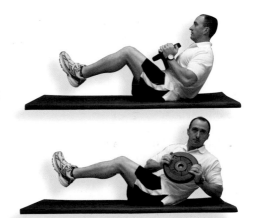

Ankle Touches (Double)

Lying down with knees bent and hands on chest. Use your abdominals to lift your shoulder blades off the ground as you extend both hands towards your left foot. Slowly return to starting position.

Tip: Squeeze shoulder coming forward to opposite hip to maximise contraction!

Grade: 2 **Low Reps:** 10 **High Reps:** 50

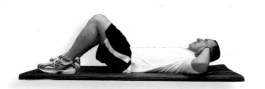

Ankle Touches (Single)

Lying down with knees bent and hands behind head (elbows out of sight). Use your abdominals to lift your shoulder blades off the ground as you extend your left hand towards your left foot. Slowly return to starting position.

Tip: Squeeze shoulder towards your hip to maximise contraction.

Grade: 1 **Low Reps:** 10 **High Reps:** 50

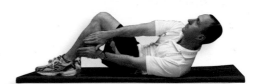

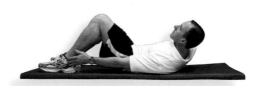

PART 3: TRAINING LIKE A WINNER

Reverse Crunch (Legs Up)

Legs straight with a 90 degree bend at the hips. Use your abdominals to push your toes upwards by pulling your pelvis towards your ribs. Do not allow your toes to come forward. Slowly lower your hips to starting position.

Tip: The only joint movement should be at the hips.

Grade: 1   **Low Reps:** 10   **High Reps:** 20

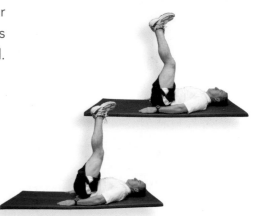

Lower back exercises

Keep movements slow and controlled to avoid injury.

Alternate Arm and Leg Raises (1st)

Lay face down on the floor with legs and arms straight. Slowly raise right arm and left leg together. Pause then lower. Repeat with left arm and right leg.

Grade: 1   **Low Reps:** 8   **High Reps:** 20

Hip Extension

Kneel on ground with hands under shoulders and back straight. Lift leg up, moving only at the hip. Only work to a range that still enables you to maintain the straight back position. Pause, then return to start position.

Grade: 1   **Low Reps:** 8   **High Reps:** 20

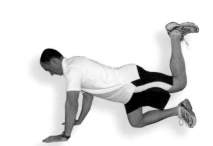

Hip Extension (with Arm)

Kneel on ground with hands under shoulders and back straight. Slowly lift opposite arm and leg up together. Only work to a range that still enables you to maintain the straight back position. Pause, then return to start position.

Grade: 1   **Low Reps:** 8   **High Reps:** 20

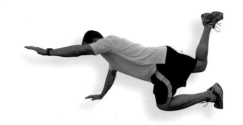

Body weight exercises

Dips

Place your hands slightly wider than shoulder width on the chair. Have your knees bent at 90 degrees. Slowly lower yourself down, then back up again. Make it harder by straightening your legs, or even putting them up on another chair.

Grade: 1   **Low Reps:** 5   **High Reps:** 20

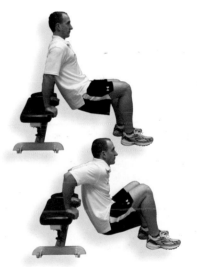

Elbows to Knee

Lift your right knee up, twist your body and touch it with your left elbows.

Grade: 1   **Low Reps:** 10   **High Reps:** 50

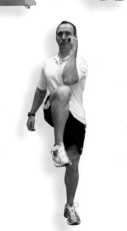

Front Punches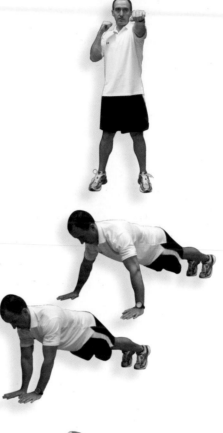

Stand with feet hip-width apart. Continuously punch out in front at shoulder level. Keep your elbows soft so you don't hyperextend.

Grade: 1   **Low Reps:** 20   **High Reps:** 100

Hand Walk

Get down into the full push up position but with your hands close together. Keeping your body straight, take one hand step out to each side, then bring them both back in again. Decrease the intensity by placing the knees on the floor, or use the wall.

Grade: 2   **Low Reps:** 8   **High Reps:** 30

High Steps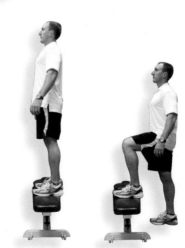

Using a chair between 20–30cm high, step up alternating between your right and left leg. When you step up onto the bench or chair, be sure to place your whole foot down so that you don't slip or trip over. If your chair is the right height, your knee should be bent at 90 degrees when you step up.

Grade: 2   **Low Reps:** 10   **High Reps:** 30

Knee Lifts

Lift each knee alternatively, up to hip level. Keep your back straight.

Grade: 1 **Low Reps:** 10 **High Reps:** 60

Lunges

Start with your feet hip-width apart, and step out to the front. Step in line with your foot's starting position. Lower down, keeping your upper body straight, then rise up. If your knee goes past your toes then you haven't taken a big enough step. Repeat on other side.

Grade: 2 **Low Reps:** 10 **High Reps:** 40

Mountain Climbers

Start with your hands shoulder-width apart. Drive your legs back and forward, bringing your front leg well forward and your back leg straight. As you tire you'll be tempted to shorten the range so be sure to maintain good form.

Grade: 3 **Low Reps:** 20 **High Reps:** 60

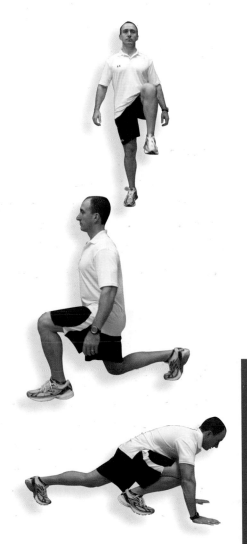

Pulsing Squats

Feet hip-width apart, with your knees going over your toes. Go down so that your thighs are parallel with the floor, then just pulse (move back and forth through a short range).

Grade: 2   **Low Reps:** 10   **High Reps:** 30

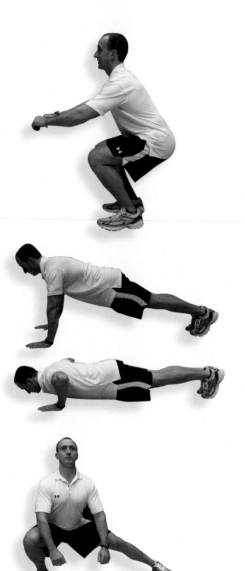

Push-ups

Place hands shoulder-width apart. On your knees for beginners or up on the toes for advanced. Keep your body flat, and neck in line with the spine. Slowly lower yourself down, then back up again.

Grade: 2   **Low Reps:** 5   **High Reps:** 30

Side Lunges

Step out to the right, and lower down, then back up again. Try to keep your upper body straight. Repeat with the left.

Grade: 3   **Low Reps:** 10   **High Reps:** 30

Squats

Feet hip-width apart, with your knees going over your toes. Try to go down so that your thighs are parallel with the floor. Try to keep your heels on the floor. If you have a knee injury or if you find it too hard to go down that low just shorten the range.

Grade: 1 **Low Reps:** 10 **High Reps:** 50

Star Jumps

Starting with your feet together and arms by your side. Jump with your feet out wide and lifting your arms up at the same time. Reduce the intensity by just using the legs, or just lifting the elbows.

Grade: 3 **Low Reps:** 10 **High Reps:** 50

Static Lunges

Start with your feet hip-width apart, and step out to the front. Lower down, then hold. Ensure that you're breathing well at all times.

Grade: 1 **Low Reps:** 20 seconds **High Reps:** 60 seconds

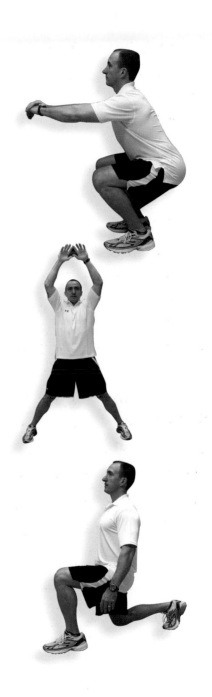

Static Squats

Start with your feet hip-width apart. Lower down so that your thighs are parallel to the floor, then hold. Ensure that you're breathing well at all times.

Grade: 1   **Low Reps:** 20 seconds   **High Reps:** 60 seconds

Wall Push-Ups (1st)

Lean against the wall with your hands shoulder-width apart, and your feet together. Keeping your body straight, lower yourself toward the wall, then press back to the starting position.

Grade: 1   **Low Reps:** 10   **High Reps:** 60

Wide Knee Lifts (1st)

Start with feet wide apart. Lift right leg up high, then left.

Grade: 1   **Low Reps:** 10   **High Reps:** 60

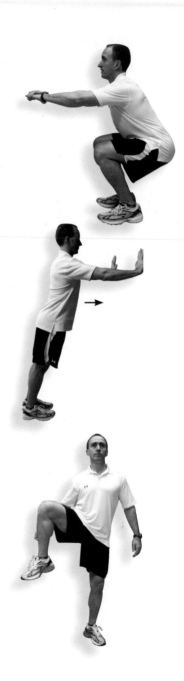

Wide Squats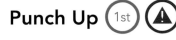

Start with your feet wide apart, with your toes pointing out. Try to go down so that your thighs are parallel with the floor, then raise up to starting position. If you have a knee injury or if you find it too hard to go down that low just shorten the range.

Grade: 1 **Low Reps:** 10 **High Reps:** 50

Punch Up (1st) ⚠

Stand with feet hip-width apart. Continuously punch above your head. Keep elbows soft.

Grade: 1 **Low Reps:** 20 **High Reps:** 100

Lateral High Steps   ⚠

Using a chair between 20–30cm high, step up laterally (sideways). When you step up onto the bench or chair, be sure to place your whole foot down so that you don't slip or trip over.

Grade: 3 **Low Reps:** 10 **High Reps:** 30

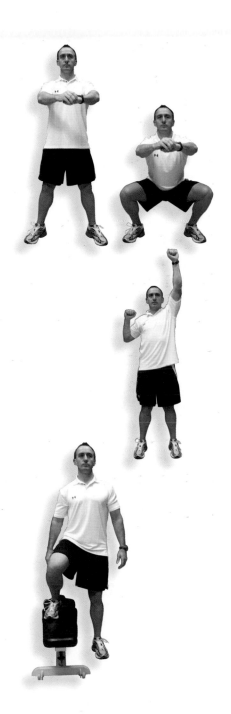

Push-ups (Feet up)

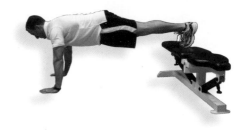

Position body so that hands are shoulder-width apart on the ground—arms fully extended, feet are together and on the toes. Keeping body flat, lower so that nose comes to the ground. Push up to start position.

Grade: 3 **Low Reps:** 10 **High Reps:** 30

Push-ups (Knees)

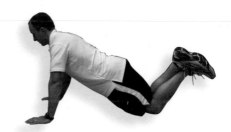

Position body so that hands are shoulder-width apart on the ground—arms fully extended, feet are together and on the toes. Keeping body flat, lower so that nose comes to the ground. Push up to start position.

Grade: 1 **Low Reps:** 10 **High Reps:** 50

Push-ups (Staggered)

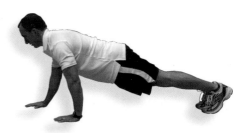

Position body so that hands are staggered, arms fully extended, feet are together and on the toes. Keeping body flat, lower so that nose comes to the ground. Push up to start position. Hands can be staggered or one hand placed on a step to focus on one side of the chest.

Grade: 3 **Low Reps:** 10 **High Reps:** 30

Plyometrics exercises

Plyometric exercises are vigorous exercises used to develop muscular power and are used to develop the force of muscular contractions, to increase the height of a jump or speed of a punch.

- Always exercise on a firm non-slip surface, and clear all obstacles out of the way
- Increase the intensity of each exercise by increasing the speed at which it's done
- Always try to land lightly

Ankle Hops

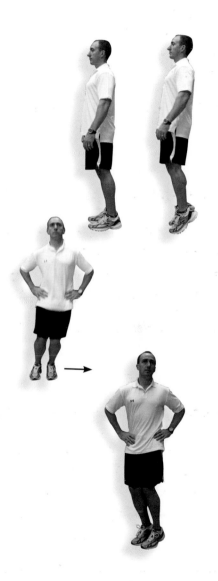

Starting with your feet flat, bounce up onto the balls of your feet, and back down again. Keep your legs straight.

Grade: 1   **Low Reps:** 10   **High Reps:** 50

Side-to-Side Ankle Hops

Keeping the legs straight, bounce from side-to-side using the ankles. When starting out just cover a short range. Increase the speed and distance as your coordination improves.

Grade: 1   **Low Reps:** 10   **High Reps:** 30

Twisting Ankle Hops

Turning the feet to the left, then the right, twisting at the hips. Keep your legs straight.

Grade: 1   **Low Reps:** 10   **High Reps:** 50

90 Degree Jumps

Starting with your feet together, jump up, turning 90 degrees before landing. Increase the intensity by jumping higher.

Grade: 2   **Low Reps:** 8   **High Reps:** 20

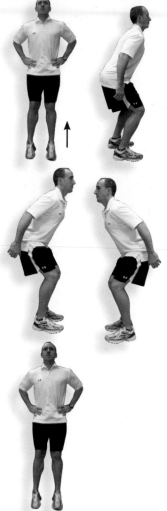

180 Degree Jumps

Jump up, turning 180 degrees in the air before landing. Increase the intensity by jumping higher.

Grade: 3   **Low Reps:** 8   **High Reps:** 20

Cross Jumps

Jumping forward, then back to the centre, left then back to the centre, back then forward to the centre, then right and back to the centre (ie North, West, South, then East).

Grade: 3   **Low Reps:** 2   **High Reps:** 10

Crouch Jumps

Keeping in a crouch position and jump up, turning 90 degrees before landing. Keep the thighs parallel to the floor.

Grade: 2   **Low Reps:** 10   **High Reps:** 30

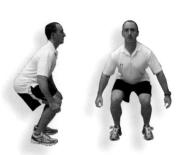

Front Toe Taps

Using a light bouncing action, tap your toes out to the front. Keep your hands on your hips, and bodyweight on your back foot.

Grade: 1   **Low Reps:** 10   **High Reps:** 50

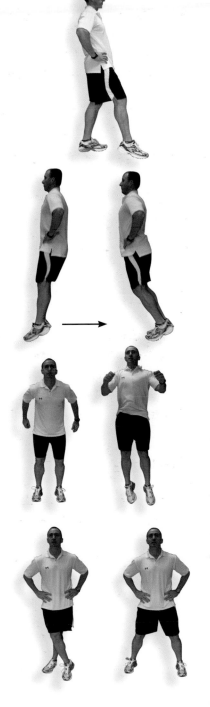

Forward/Back Ankle Hops

Keeping the legs straight, bounce from front-to-back using the ankles. Increase the intensity by jumping longer.

Grade: 2   **Low Reps:** 8   **High Reps:** 20

Lateral Jumps

In the one action, take a quick dip down, swing the arms, and jump sideways. Increase the intensity by jumping higher.

Grade: 2   **Low Reps:** 8   **High Reps:** 20

Lateral Scissor Jumps

Starting with your legs wide, cross them over, then back again. Keep the movement non-stop.

Grade: 1   **Low Reps:** 10   **High Reps:** 3

Long Jumps

In the one action, take a quick dip down, swing the arms, and jump as far as you can. Turn around, and go back. Do this on a firm surface. If you do it on a rug or mat you may slip over.

Grade: 3   **Low Reps:** 8   **High Reps:** 20

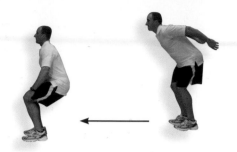

Scissor Jumps

Start with one leg out in front and the other back. Jump up and swap them over.

Grade: 1   **Low Reps:** 10   **High Reps:** 50

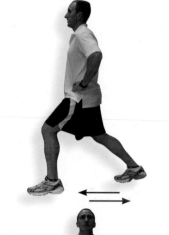

Side Toe Taps

Using a light bouncing action, tap your toes out to the side. Keep your hands on your hips.

Grade: 1   **Low Reps:** 10   **High Reps:** 50

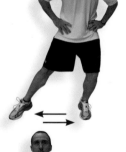

Ski Tuck Jumps

Start in a crouched position with your feet wide. Jump up and bring your feet in, then jump again and take them out wide again. Keep your thighs parallel to the floor.

Grade: 2   **Low Reps:** 10   **High Reps:** 30

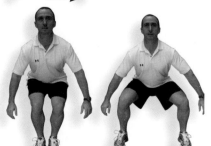

Squat Jumps

Place your hands on your head, squat down, then jump up as high as you can.

Grade: 2   **Low Reps:** 8   **High Reps:** 20

Straight Leg Bounds

Leaning back slightly, kick your legs out to the front. Stay on the balls of your feet, and keep your legs straight. Increase the intensity by kicking your legs higher.

Grade: 3   **Low Reps:** 10   **High Reps:** 50

Vertical Jumps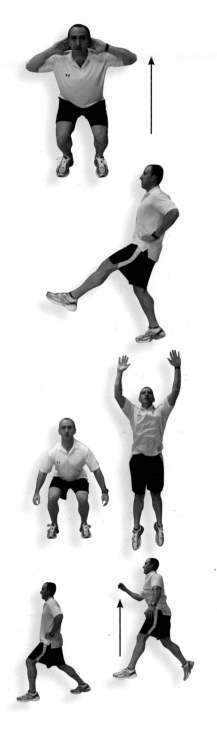

In the one action, take a quick dip down, swing the arms, and jump up as high as you can.

Grade: 2   **Low Reps:** 8   **High Reps:** 20

Lunge Jumps

Start with one leg out in front and the other back. Jump up high, and swap them over.

Grade: 3   **Low Reps:** 8   **High Reps:** 20

Cardio exercises

Make sure that you keep your heart rate over 120 bpm.

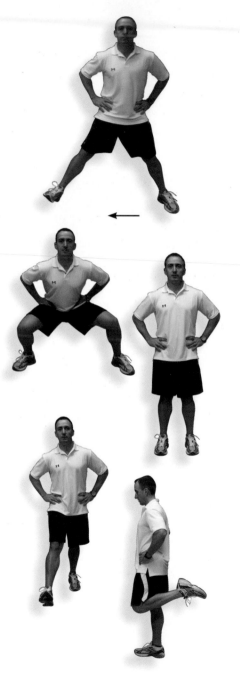

2 Steps-Side (1st)

Take 2 steps to the left, then 2 to the right. Increase the intensity by adding a little skip between the steps.

Grade: 1 **Low Reps:** 30 seconds **High Reps:** 60 seconds

Duck-Side (1st)

Take a big step to the side, ducking down as you move, then back up. Keep body straight. Hands on hips.

Grade: 1 **Low Reps:** 30 seconds **High Reps:** 60 seconds

Front Steps (1st)

Take a step to the front and then back again. Increase intensity by clapping above head when out in front.

Grade: 1 **Low Reps:** 30 seconds **High Reps:** 60 seconds

Heel Flicks (1st)

Lift your heels up lightly, one foot at a time.

Grade: 1 **Low Reps:** 30 seconds **High Reps:** 60 seconds

Heel Taps

Tap heels out to the front alternating between right and left. Hands on hips for beginners or push hands out to front to increase the intensity.

Grade: 1 **Low Reps:** 30 seconds **High Reps:** 60 seconds

High Knee Runs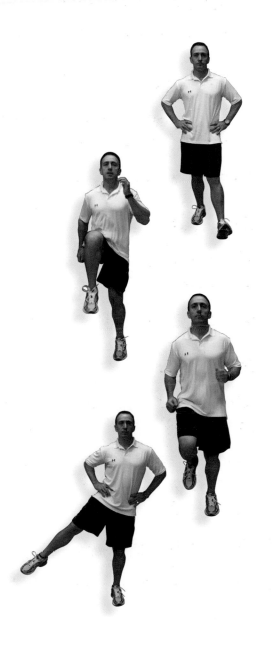

Lift knees high. Keep body straight. Pump your arms. Try to land lightly.

Grade: 3 **Low Reps:** 20 seconds **High Reps:** 60 seconds

Jog

Slow for beginners. Jog faster if you feel you can go harder. Move your arms. Try to land lightly.

Grade: 2 **Low Reps:** 30 seconds **High Reps:** 60 seconds

Side Flicks

Lifting your leg to the side and flicking your foot out lightly. Lift your leg higher to increase the intensity.

Grade: 1 **Low Reps:** 30 seconds **High Reps:** 60 seconds

Side Steps

Step from side to side. If you'd like to burn more calories add a clap out in front each time you step.

Grade: 1   **Low Reps:** 30 seconds   **High Reps:** 60 seconds

Side Taps

Tap toes to the side. Hands on hips or if you'd like more of a challenge add some arm raises.

Grade: 1   **Low Reps:** 30 seconds   **High Reps:** 60 seconds

Skates

Step side to side like you are skating. Lean forward and take big steps. Increase the intensity by increasing the pace and size of steps.

Grade: 3   **Low Reps:** 30 seconds   **High Reps:** 60 seconds

Skipping

This is especially good for those who keep getting the rope wrapped around their feet. Lightly jump up and down landing on both feet. Keep your knees slightly bent when landing to absorb the impact. At the same time, make the hands do small circles as though you're turning your rope. Remember to land as lightly as possible.

Grade: 2   **Low Reps:** 30 seconds   **High Reps:** 60 seconds

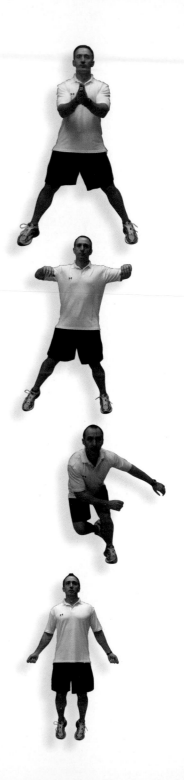

Step Knee Lift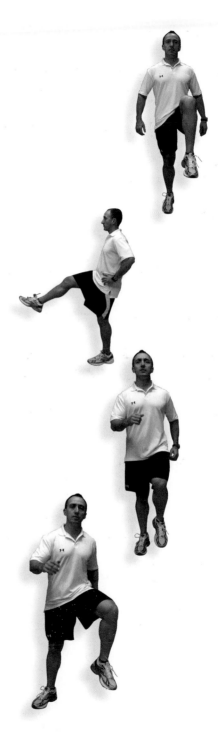

Take a step out to the front with the left leg, then lift the right knee. Step back to starting position. Repeat with the left side. Increase the intensity by adding a little hop as you lift the knee.

Grade: 2 **Low Reps:** 30 seconds **High Reps:** 60 seconds

Toe Kicks (1st)

Lifting your knee up and lightly flicking your foot to the front. Lift your leg higher to increase the intensity. Alternate each leg.

Grade: 1 **Low Reps:** 30 seconds **High Reps:** 60 seconds

Walk (1st)

Pump arms. Walk fast if you're an experienced exerciser or just go steady if you're just starting out.

Grade: 1 **Low Reps:** 30 seconds **High Reps:** 60 seconds

Wide Walks (1st)

Walk with your feet out wide. Toes slightly pointing out. Lift your leg higher to increase the intensity.

Grade: 1 **Low Reps:** 30 seconds **High Reps:** 60 seconds

Boxing exercises

Starting Position:

- Stand with your feet hip width apart
- Take a step forward with the left foot
- Place the back foot at a 45 degree angle
- Keep body weight on the balls of the feet.
- Keep the knees bent
- Place your right hand up near your right cheek, and your left hand at the same height but slightly out in front
- Keep your chin down and elbows into the ribs
- Turn your shoulders so that your left shoulder is ahead of your right
- * Reverse each of these instructions if you are left-handed

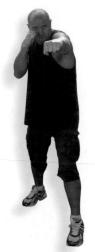

The Jab

Pushing off the back foot, throw a straight punch with the left hand at chin level. Rotate hand as it leaves your chin. Fully clench fist just before impact. Return to start position.

Right Hook

Transfer body weight to the right side. Bring right elbow up so that it is parallel with the floor, elbow is bent at 90 degrees.

Pivot on the right foot, turning the right leg and torso.

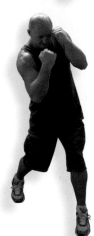

Left Hook

Transfer body weight to the left side. Bring left elbow up so that it is parallel with the floor, elbow is bent at 90 degrees. Pivot on the left foot, turning the left leg and torso.

Straight Right

Starting with your hand next to your cheek, punch in a straight line at chin level The punch starts at the feet, so push off your back foot, then rotate your hips, rotate the shoulders, and follow through with the punch. Body weight should remain centred, so don't lean forward too far as this will place you off balance.

Left Uppercut

Transfer body weight to the left side. Dip left hip and shoulder. Drive punch straight up, pushing off left foot.

Right Uppercut

Transfer body weight to the right side. Dip right hip and shoulder. Drive punch straight up, pushing off right foot.

Left to the Body

Drop left hand. Rotate the left leg and torso sharply. Drive punch in at lower rib level.

Right to the Body

Drop right hand. Rotate the right leg and torso sharply. Drive punch in at lower rib level.

Boxing combinations:

You can choose any combination for each boxing station on the circuit:

Left Jab

Double Jab

Triple Jab

Straight Right

Left Hook

Right Hook

Left Uppercut

Right Uppercut

Double Jab–Straight Right

Jab High–Jab Low

Jab–Straight Right

Jab–Straight Right–Left Hook

Left Hook–Straight Right–Left Hook

Left Uppercut–Straight Right

Right Body–Left Hook

Right Hook–Left Hook

Left Hook–Right Hook

Right Uppercut–Left Hook

Straight Right–Left Hook

Straight Right–Left Hook–Straight Right

Triple Jab–Straight Right

Jab–Straight Right–Duck–Straight Right

Jab–Duck–Straight Right

Jab–Straight Right–Duck–Right Uppercut

Stretches

Abdominal

Lay face down on the ground with your body weight supported on your hands or elbows. Lift head up and push abdominals toward the floor.

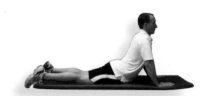

Chest 1

Join hands together behind the back. Maintaining an upright position, lift the hands up (keep your arms straight).

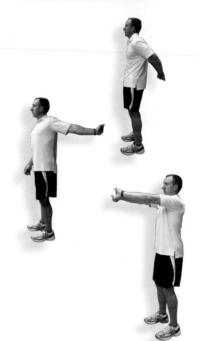

Chest 2

Place your hand on a wall or pole at shoulder level. Turn your shoulders away until you feel the stretch.

Front Stretch

Join hands together and turn palms away from your body. Round your back and push away from your body with your hands.

Tricep

Place your hand behind your head with your elbows pointing up. Place your other hand on your elbows and gently pull towards your left arm (you can also lean to the side to extend the stretch throughout your body).

Groin

Take a big step out to the front. Make sure your hips are square, tuck pelvis and push hips forward.

Standing Quadricep

Pull your foot towards your butt. Keep your knees together and push your hips forwards (you can hold onto a wall if you have trouble balancing).

Soleus

Make sure your toes are in line with your knee. Keep your heel on the ground. Place body weight on top of thigh. Lean forward until you feel the stretch.

Shoulder

Bring your arm across your body at shoulder height. Use your other arm to pull towards your body.

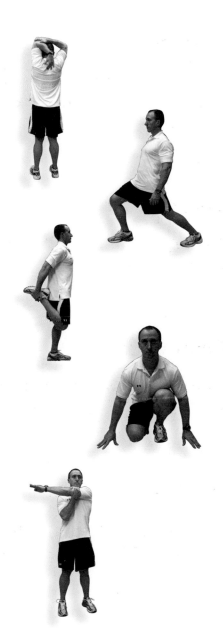

Overhead Push

Join your hands together. Standing up straight, raise your arms above your head with palms facing upwards, push away from your body.

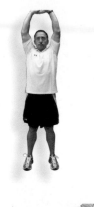

Lying Quad

Lying face down, bend leg. Reach hand behind back, grasp foot and pull towards your bottom. Push your hips into the floor.

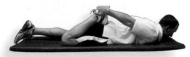

Seated Hamstring

Sit with one leg out to the front, and the other leg bent. Keeping your back straight, lean forward until you feel the stretch along your hamstring.

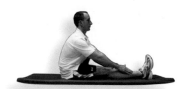

Standing Calf

Stand with one foot forward, with your back leg bent. Place all your body weight on the back leg.

Standing Hamstring

Place your heel into the floor. Keeping the back straight, bend forward until you feel the stretch.

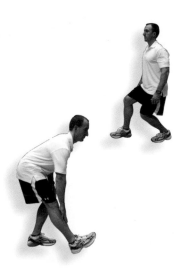

Twisting Stretch

Sit with one leg out to the front, and the other leg bent. Place the bent leg on the other side of the straight leg. Turn the upper body around, placing the opposite arm against the bent leg.

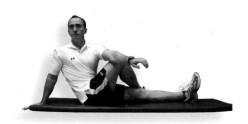

PART FOUR: WINNING TIPS

Think about your everyday life for a moment: How often do things go according to plan? Rarely. Inconveniences, work commitments, personal struggles (general life!) just get in the way. The same is true of a weight loss program. Blowing your diet one day or not finding time to exercise is not a failure, rather an expectation of daily life, so you can't give in over one chocolate bar or week of no exercise! Those who win their weight loss journey are not those who never encounter an obstacle, but those who see an obstacle as a challenge and do the necessary work to climb over it. To help you overcome the common challenges that pop up when trying to eat better, exercise and lose weight, read on …

18. Diet troubleshooting

As any dieter will tell you, things rarely go as planned. Your willpower buckles at the smell of freshly baked bread. You couldn't possibly be rude by turning down an offering of dessert. That chocolate bar at the checkout really did call out 'Eat me!' You really did intend to stick to your diet but you had a stressful week. You tried to eat well but they didn't have any healthy food at the party you went to.

Let's be honest, with so many food temptations around us 24/7 it would be unrealistic to expect anyone to not veer off the diet road from time to time! But what determines success is whether or not your diet detour is a simple wrong turn, which you can fix by getting back on the right road, or a detour that leads you down the path to diet destruction: a full-blown crash, bang, binge!

Bouncing back from a binge

You can't let a binge be a reason to say, 'Well, I've blown it now, I may as well keep eating'. Instead, see it as a learning experience by tracing things back to the source of the binge. Was it poor planning, emotions getting the better of you, or just a plain what-the-heck-I'm-going-to-indulge moment? Learn where it came from and do better next time you feel a similar binge come over you.

Binge busters

The reasons we binge are varied. I recently had a patient who really struggled with bingeing and couldn't work out why. Below are the steps of deduction I went through with him to find a solution to his impulsive bingeing. In the end, the only thing that worked was getting him away from his everyday distractions. If you're having trouble with repeated bingeing, get to the source of the problem and come up with a solution:

- Are you getting enough carbohydrates? Stock up on some extra unrefined complex carbohydrates. Quite often, low energy levels trigger bingeing as your body craves masses of food to bring its energy levels up fast.

- Are you eating too many simple carbohydrates? Stock up on more lean protein as it helps stabilise blood sugar.

- Are you waiting for too long between meals? Your blood sugar levels drop when you wait too long. Eat a small meal at least every three hours.

- Are you bored? Try exercising at the time you commonly binge.

- Are you not thinking about what you're eating? Snacking in front of the TV, eating at parties and social functions, and eating too quickly can see you eating too much without even realising it. Eat slowly, chewing every mouthful around 20 times and keep your mind in the moment of eating, tasting and appreciating every mouthful.

- Are you dehydrated? Be sure you're getting your eight glasses of water—more if you're exercising. The body can mistakenly crave food when it's really thirsty.

- Are you emotional? A big binge can actually have a sedative effect, helping you feel calm and offering a temporary state of relief and contentment. Find other ways to deal with your emotions. See 'Tips for beating emotional eating' in Chapter 9 for coping strategies.

- Are you drinking too much? Alcohol can increase our desire for salty, fatty foods. Keep alcohol to a minimum and never drink on an empty stomach.

Trade-offs

If you overdo it with one meal by eating too many calories, you can exercise off the excess calories. For example, a person who weighs 70 kilograms (154 pounds) who eats half a 250 gram (8 oz) block of cheese (500 calories) needs to do an extra 41 minutes of running. Below are some other examples of how to burn off foods of a similar calorie content:

How alcohol hinders weight loss

Alcohol has a high calorie and sugar content.

Extra calories consumed because you're more likely to eat poorly (the 2am hot dog or kebab!)

Your body is too busy burning up the sugar alcohol contains, so you're not giving it a chance to burn its fat stores.

Alcohol is a diuretic; you'll lose fluid, minerals, and electrolytes. This will throw off your training as you're less likely to train the next day, and even if you do the quality is usually poor.

4 cans of beer =	114 minutes x walking
2 plain donuts =	51 minutes x cycling
1 medium block =	62 minutes x swimming laps (freestyle) chocolate
100 gram packet =	68 minutes x boxing (bag) potato chips
1 Big Mac =	64 minutes x hard weight-training
1.25 litre bottle cola =	54 minutes x circuit training

Dealing with special occasions

You may be trying to lose weight, but that doesn't mean you can't socialise. Cutting loose every weekend will surely bring you undone but if you plan for it you can have a great time at the occasions that are special to you. However, we need to stop including everyone else's special occasions in with our own. To be successful with weight loss you need to sacrifice the less important events to enjoy the more important ones. You need to work out which occasions are most important to you.

Planning for special occasions

Sit down and write the dates of the events that mean the most to you in your Weight Loss Journal or on the Pay-it-Forward Planner in the Appendix. This could be your birthday, your partner's birthday, wedding anniversary, and Christmas. You could add a few others if you wish, but for most people these are the main ones. For these you may allow for a big increase of calories on that day (1500–2000 extra). For any other events only allow for a small increase (400–500 extra). You shouldn't usually have any more than 12 (one per month) special events throughout the year. If you do, you may have to look a bit closer at what you find important.

If you plan ahead you'll be able to enjoy the extra food and alcohol, without the guilt. For each special occasion work out how many drinks you wish to have and how many calories worth of food.

Here's the catch: you'll have to pay it back in training! Only instead of doing the damage and then making up for it by burning it off and/or restricting your calories, you're going to pay it forward!

Pay it forward

As long as you're following one of our calorie-controlled eating plans you will be able to allow up to an extra 1800 calories for the day. This isn't hard to get to. For example:

½ bottle wine = approximately 280 calories

3 course dinner = approximately 1600 calories

How many times have you buckled under pressure as you arrive at a dinner party and say yes to fried finger food as an appetiser and a glass of champagne? Then tell yourself that it's okay, 'I'll just work it off at the gym on Monday' or 'I'll eat good on Monday to make up for it'? But Monday comes and you forget about your little pay-it-back promise or simply can't be bothered. Whatever the reason, you just don't get around to making up for those excess calories you consumed at that dinner party.

By planning for each big occasion, at least four weeks in advance, you'll be able to burn the extra calories in advance without much trouble.

Example 1: A person who walks briskly (4 METS) for 60 minutes each day.

To share an extra 1800 calories over 28 days (4 weeks), means you have to burn an extra 64 calories in each session. If you weigh 80 kilograms (176 pounds), for example, you'll need to walk an extra 12 minutes each day. If you're 100 kilograms (220 pounds), for example, you'll need to walk 11 minutes extra each session. See Chapter 7 for how to calculate this.

For example 2: A person who runs (8 METS) for 60 minutes each day.

To share an extra 1800 calories over 28 days (4 weeks), means an 80 kilograms (176 pounds) person will have to run an extra 6 minutes, whilst a 100 kilograms (220 pounds) runner would have to do an extra 5 minutes each day.

Note: Visit the Pay-it-Forward calculator at *www.raykellyfitness.com*

Set up a plan for the next three months of special occasions (I'm sure there will be more than one!).

List the amount of extra calories you'd like to consume on those days and then include a plan of how you will make those calories up before that time. You can do this in your Weight Loss Journal, or on the Pay-it-Forward Planner (see Appendix)

Didn't pay it forward? You can still pay it back, by adding up the calories you didn't plan to eat, or didn't burn in advance, and burn them off after the episode. See examples of trade-offs in Chapter 18.

Other special occasion strategies

Try an active catch-up: Instead of catching up for dinner, coffee and cake or drinks, why not catch up for a social game of golf or tennis, a walk-and-talk with your friend/s, or kicking a soccer ball, playing touch footy or a game of cricket in the park followed by a picnic packed with healthy food.

Coping with Christmas: You'll need to have some strategies in place to ensure you don't overindulge. And make sure you are exercising every day—even if all you can manage is more walking around doing Christmas shopping! Only go over your prescribed calorie intake on the big celebration days such as Christmas day.

Eat before a party: By turning up to a party with your stomach full, you'll be less likely to pick on 'danger' finger foods, such as party pies! Otherwise, opt for the healthier versions, such as carrots and celery sticks with hommus dip.

Watch what you drink: If you want to enjoy an alcoholic drink, some tips to keep the calorie content down: drink two glasses of water in between every drink; make one glass last by sipping slowly, so you still look like you're being part of the festivities by having a drink in your hand; don't let someone fill your glass before you're finished, as it's too easy to lose track of how much you've really had; and opt for lower calorie containing alcohol such as vodka, fresh lime and soda instead of wine or a low-carb beer instead of a full-strength beer.

Volunteer as the designated driver: If you feel that your willpower may be low, volunteer as the designated driver so others are relying on you not to drink.

Overcome peer pressure: Some people just can't take no for an answer, so if you feel that you won't be able to survive the constant peer pressure of the night, try a few white lies to help your cause: 'I can't drink because I'm on antibiotics'; 'I can't eat because I haven't been able to keep food down' or something along these lines.

Take a friend for support: Take a reliable friend who is also trying to lose weight for that extra bit of support. You can keep each other honest!

Tips for eating out

You may think that the only way you can keep to your diet is to lock yourself inside and never venture out. With some clever choices you can enjoy eating out without worrying about damaging side effects.

- Avoid going out to dinner starving. If you do turn up ravenous, ask for a small bowl of soup (no butter or cream) or a green salad to tide you over before your main meal, instead of picking at bread.

- Never order anything that is fried. Go for steamed, poached or grilled/broiled.

- Don't trust the term 'grilled' straight off as it can be coated with butter or olive oil and cooked on top of a hot plate. This is common with 'grilled fish'.

- Be wary of stir-fry's. Although they are the healthier option some places can overdo it with the oil, so ask for just a little oil or no oil.

- Ask for no butter or cream to be added to your food. If you feel self conscious about going to so much trouble tell them that you're allergic to dairy and it makes you horribly sick.

- Stock up on salad and vegetables for side dishes instead of chips or mashed potato.

- Share your dessert or ask for some fresh fruit.

- To keep the overall calorie content down: if you want to have dessert, choose an entrée as your main meal; if you just want one meal choose a main meal; if you want two meals choose two entrée-sized meals as your entrée and your main.

- Eat slowly, enjoy your dinner company, put your knife and fork down regularly between bites and slowly sip on one glass of wine or mineral water. The longer you drag out your meal the less chance of overeating.

- Go to a café that has 'wholefoods' or you know cook with all-natural ingredients.

- Meet for breakfast or brunch instead of dinner or lunch; that way alcohol won't be involved and you can enjoy something healthy such as poached eggs, spinach, and baked beans on wholegrain toast—hold the butter. Choose bacon and lean sausages only sometimes as an extra special treat. Skip the hash browns and pancakes!

- Opt for tomato-based sauces and not creamy sauces when eating Italian.

- Skip the curries and hold the rice to save calories when eating Asian.

- If you have no other options but fast food, Subway is a great choice or order a burger (no fries) and eat the meat and salad only.

- Fish (not battered or fried or covered in butter-based sauce) with salad or vegetables is usually the safest choice in any restaurant.

- Squeeze lemon juice over your salad instead of oil dressing.

- Get any sauces or dressings on a side plate so you can add your own. This way you can control how much goes on.

- If salad or vegies come with the meal eat them first so you won't have to fill up on the higher calorie foods.

- Avoid all buffets!

- It may not be always on the menu but most restaurants will be able to provide you with a healthy fruit salad for dessert. Just ask.

- Trim the visible fat off meat.

- Put half your main meal aside to take home.

19. Exercise troubleshooting

So things are going well, you're sticking to your exercise program but then something happens to get you off the exercise track: perhaps it's an injury; you have less time to workout; or you're not getting results, despite your hard work, and you're feeling fed up! Don't let an exercise derailment send you back to the couch.

When your workout isn't working out

- Finding you're regularly skipping workouts? Try a new activity you find more enjoyable.

- Finding it hard to make time to exercise? Break your workouts up into several smaller sessions over the day.

- Are your legs feeling like lead? Switch to boxing for your cardio sessions to give your legs a rest.

- Muscle soreness not going away? Allow a good 48–72 hours in between weight-training sessions and include some rest days.

- Despite having the best intentions you just can't get motivated to exercise? Find a training partner or exercise group, hire a personal trainer or simply do more incidental activity.

- Don't have the energy to make it through a good workout? You may need to have a light snack, such as a piece of fruit, within an hour of starting your workout. Also be sure to eat a well-balanced meal within two hours of finishing your workout to help replenish glycogen stores and help you recover for your next session. Sports dieticians say refuelling in the first 30–60 minutes post-workout is optimal.

- Are you bored with your exercise sessions? Might be time to try more challenging workouts or changing your workout routine altogether.

- The weights you once lifted are now easy? You need to increase the intensity by increasing the reps, sets or weight.

- Is boredom a factor? Try shorter, more intense sessions. Sometimes we get caught up in the duration of our training and we forget how important training quality is. Throw in a few sessions each week where you only train for 20 minutes, but at a much higher intensity. Interval training is great for this!

- Losing exercise inspiration? Change your training environment. Train indoors, outdoors, or at another fitness centre. Changing your environment can really freshen your training.

Rest and recovery

Recovery forms an integral part of every training regime. It provides the body with the optimum environment for the repair and rejuvenation of the body and mind. Recovery allows the body to adapt to the training program and come back at full strength. Omit recovery from your program and you are heading down the path of injury and mental fatigue!

It can come in many forms. It could be simply taking one day per week off training for total rest, having a full week of light training every 4–6 weeks, having a massage, listening to music, or a combination of all of these. The level of recovery required is based on the overall load you are placing on your body. Incorporate these R n' R tips into your routine:

Rest day: Sundays are great for this!

Recovery weeks: If you are following the progressive overload principle then you must incorporate recovery weeks to avoid injury or over-training. (The progressive overload principle is increasing your training load regularly in a step-like fashion: increase the workload once your workout is no longer challenging, allow time for your body to adapt to the increased workload, increase the workload again when it is no longer challenging and so on.) During this week don't stop doing your training program, just reduce the intensity. This is a great time to concentrate on your training technique, which will improve your performance when you get back to increased loads.

Cross training: This is participating in an activity, which is different to your normal training regime. Indoor rock-climbing, cycling, rowing, basketball, or in-line skating are just a few examples of alternative exercises to a running or walking program. This gives the muscles a break, while still maintaining some level of condition by doing an activity that works your body in different ways. The only requirement is that the intensity must be light.

Sleep: This is often what people do when they have finished everything else for that day but it must become a higher priority. A lack of sleep makes people irrational, moody, and low on energy. Try to get seven to nine hours sleep per night. To ensure a great night's sleep avoid alcohol, caffeine, nicotine and high protein meals late at night.

Hot/cold shower: Never do this if you are suffering from a virus or cold or if you have a recent soft tissue injury. This method involves alternating the water temperature between hot and cold for set periods, which has been shown to increase the blood flow to the working muscles and help rid lactic acid from the muscles. Start by having a shower with the water at the usual temperature and clean your skin with soap. The temperature is then alternated between hot for 1–2 minutes, then cold for 10–30 seconds. Repeat this three times then shower and re-hydrate to finish.

Hot/cold spa: Guidelines are the same as for the hot/cold shower but 3–4 minutes is spent in the spa and 30–60 seconds is spent in the cold bath.

Massage: A great way to promote recovery because it increases blood flow deep into the muscles, and is really relaxing! Swedish massage is generally the lightest form but some people really like a deep tissue massage. Be sure to only consult a suitably qualified and registered massage therapist.

Meditation: This has immense benefits for relaxation and healing. Join a local meditation group or buy one of the many instructional CDs on the market. Meditate in an environment that is comfortable and with minimal noise and distractions. You may find yourself falling asleep the first few times you try this but it is a great way of relaxing and also provides you with greater concentration skills. You can even visualise a slimmer you while you're in your state of Zen!

Progressive muscle relaxation: This is a simple way of relaxing the mind with minimal expense or training. Start by lying on the floor, on your back with your hands by your side, and your eyes closed. Imagine you are at the most relaxing place you could imagine—it may include a tropical island, waterfalls, whatever you find relaxing. Whilst you are thinking about the sight, smell, and sounds of your surrounding take 20 long, deep breaths. Once you've reached 20 you will be ready to begin the muscle relaxation. Start at the toes by tightening (contracting) the muscles in the toes for 5 seconds then relax them. As you relax them feel the tension sink from those muscles and escape the body into the ground. Work your way slowly through the body going to the feet, calves, upper thigh, abdominals, hands, arms, chest, shoulders, neck, and then the face. Each time feeling the body sink deeper into the floor as the tension is released from your muscles. Finish with 10 more deep breaths.

Music: Just kick back, relax, and listen to any music that you enjoy. You will be surprised at how mentally refreshing this can be!

Movies: Go and watch a new movie at the cinema or hire out one of your favourites from the DVD store. Once again, a great way to relieve stress and relax mentally!

Training with injury

An injury doesn't have to throw your workout routine off track. You just need to be a bit more creative with your exercise planning. You can switch activities so you're still working out but not straining the injured part. For example:

- Do boxing if you have a lower limb injury

- Swim or walk if you're suffering from lower back pain

- Run or walk if you have an upper body injury

- Do an upper body weights circuit if you have a lower limb injury

- Do an abdominal and leg weights circuit if you have an upper body injury.

20. Weight loss troubleshooting

Nothing can be more frustrating than putting in the hard yards but not getting rewarded with a loss on the scales. If your weight loss isn't progressing along as you'd like, instead of getting disappointed and throwing the towel in, re-think your strategies and keep trying different things until your ideal rate of weight loss takes hold.

I'm not losing ... why?

Plateaus, are quite common, but they don't have to be. When you hit a plateau it seems that nothing will shift your weight loss out of pause mode and into play.

If your weight loss is stuck in neutral, here are some tips to get your weight loss moving again:

Get back to basics: Start measuring your food because it's easy to fool yourself into thinking that you're eating well.

Take out your Food Diary again: Be honest so you can pick problem points in your diet.

Do some calculating: Log the calories you consume for one week and the calories you burn, including metabolism (see Chapter 7) and make sure you're making a calorie deficit. If not, you may need to reduce your calorie intake or increase your exercise.

Mix up your calories: If you're counting calories, try varying the amount you have each day but keep the weekly average around the same.

Increase the intensity: It's easy to fall into your comfort zone when you haven't changed your program for a while. Quite often you'll find the reason for your plateau is that you've adapted to your program and it's no longer challenging.

Change your training days or times: Mixing up your training days or times can change the way you feel about training. Maybe your situation has changed and before you were more of a morning trainer but now you are better in the afternoons.

Change your training altogether: Starting a new type of exercise can make training interesting again. It can also bring more of a challenge, which can mean more calories burned! Instead of walking or running, try swimming, cycling, or tennis.

Chaffing

Exercising for large people can be uncomfortable due to chaffing when body bits rub together. To help with chaffing, wear natural fibres such as 100 percent cotton, wrap elastic bandaging around the bits that rub together, wear lycra bike shorts under your track pants or shorts to prevent inner thigh chaffing or try Vaseline or talcum powder on the affected areas.

Re-plan your whole life! Start from scratch. Write down your exercising and eating times and stick to it!

Are you training too much? More isn't always better so sometimes it's better to decrease the amount of exercise you're doing. Sometimes having a rest can actually get you losing weight again.

Hire a personal trainer: Even if you're knowledgeable in fitness, a different training style or someone to push you may be just what you need to get the scales moving again.

See a nutritionist or dietician: Just one session can help identify areas of your diet that are hindering your weight loss.

Try some new recipes: Grab a new cookbook and make each meal a new adventure.

Mix up your weight-training program: By changing the exercises, exercise order, reps, sets, or rest intervals. Just adjusting any one of these will change your program altogether and force your body to work harder to adjust to the changes, and burn extra calories in the process.

Find a new training partner that is fitter than you are: You'll find that you'll be training at their level in no time, which will take your calorie burning to a new level!

Are you self-sabotaging? Once you've ruled out physical factors, look to what emotional factors could be stopping you from wanting to lose weight. See Chapter 4.

You need a break: Sometimes just taking some time out for rest and relaxation or doing alternative gentle activities can do the trick of getting the scales moving again, and also to recharge your batteries for some more hard training.

Still not losing after trying all of these strategies? Speak with your doctor to rule out possible medical reasons.

21. Maintaining your weight loss

Most people will admit that with a bit of extra exercise and calorie control it's not all that hard to lose weight. What is hard is maintaining the weight you've lost. How many times have you done the yo-yo thing? Dropped weight, only to have it bounce back up (sometimes to a higher figure than before) then repeat the cycle all over again.

To make sure your weight loss sticks, try these tips:

Learn the art of trade-offs (see Chapter 18): Never let a bad week break you. Burn off any extra calories you consumed with extra exercise.

Drop the excuses: 'I was good when I had my personal trainer but now I can't afford it'; 'I need the gym to lose weight and my membership ran out'; 'I got a new job and I just didn't have the time anymore'—you know the excuses. You're worth more than some lame excuse. If you've done the hard work honour your efforts by being true to the new you! With every new challenge, there's a new solution; you just have to find it.

Find a new goal: The goal of losing weight can be your driving force, but what drives you once you've lost the weight? You need to find a new source of motivation to keep up your new healthy eating and exercise habits. This could be a fitness goal, such as running a marathon or building more muscle, or a personal goal such as going overseas and taking an empowering trek or maintaining your body to help you feel self-confident enough to find a loving partner.

Try a completely new diet: Try a different style of eating, such as Asian or Mediterranean and teach yourself how to eat healthy and stick to your calorie count within this style of cuisine.

Commit to buying a new cookbook every month: This way you've always got new ideas to keep your meals interesting.

Take up any exciting new activities: Try something you've always wanted to try but never felt fit or thin enough to do, such as rock-climbing, ballroom dancing, surfing or skiing.

Exercise is your highest priority: Once you let that slip, your eating will soon follow.

Plan to have your workouts changed regularly: Variety means that boredom doesn't creep up on you.

Join a team sport: Sport commits you to exercise for the full season.

22. Childhood Obesity

Getting Kids to Eat Healthy Foods

We all know that childhood obesity is a growing problem. We have a new generation of children that have grown up on processed foods, less activity, and parents with less time due to both having a career. Often I have parents who bring their children in to the clinic for a solution to the problem, hoping that I can motivate their child to eat healthy foods and become more active. But the problem often isn't with the child, but with the parent!

Now before you close the book and throw it across the room, just hear me out. Here are the three usual scenarios that I see happening within the home:

1. The parent notices the child's weight is increasing so the parent does the right thing and asks the child to eat healthier foods. The child refuses because all of their life they've seen their own parents screw their nose up at salads or vegetables. Think about it, there's no one in this world this child trusts more than their parents, and this is the same person who is passing them these new foods, all the while eating takeaway or processed foods themselves.

2. The parent offers the child healthy foods. The child refuses to eat it knowing full well the parent will give them what they want if they hold out. The parent eventually goes back to giving them processed foods.

3. The parent offers the child healthy foods. The child accepts. As a reward the child gets given unhealthy food as a treat so it defeats the purpose.

I'm not saying it's easy to get kids eating healthy foods but the consequences are so bad that it just has to be done. No one wants to hand their child a life of Type 2 diabetes (we are now seeing 14 year olds diagnosed), high blood pressure, polycystic ovarian syndrome, sleep apnoea, osteoarthritis, depression and low self-esteem. But today's children will be dealing with these issues in their 20's and 30's!

So what can you do?

1. **Be a role model!** Your children look up to you, so if they see you eating these foods and leading an active life there's a much greater chance that they will adopt the same.

2. **Give them choices!** Allow them to make a choice, but make sure each option is healthy. Once they have that involvement they'll be much more likely to eat it.

3. **Only give healthy choices!** If you want them to eat healthy then only give healthy options. Kids need guidance but if you offer something that is high in sugar, fat, or salt chances are they will choose that.

4. **Be strong!** Too many parents give in too easily, and the kids know it. If they are hungry they will eat! Just be sure to give them options.

5. **No open access to the cupboards/fridge!** Kids need to learn that they can't just eat whenever they like. They only need to eat every few hours. So set eating times for the three main meals a day with two to three snacks.

6. **Don't bring the bad food in to the house!** One of the biggest issues for people of any age when losing weight is the high accessibility of poor foods in their own cupboards. For kids it's even worse because in most cases it's their parents that are bringing them in (and quite often, eating it in front of them).

Ray Kelly's 4 x 1 Diet

We all know kids can be picky eaters so you need to have a flexible plan if you want to get them to eat healthy. The 4x 1 diet is something I've used with my girls with great success because they have been able to make their own food choices. The 4 x 1 Diet works like this: when you and your children walk into the fresh food section of a supermarket, let each child choose 4 of any items in that area. You will be surprised at the combinations they choose! We often see a plate that could contain raw broccoli, grapes, zucchini and peach. If they get to choose what they eat themselves, then you have a greater chance of them eating it.

If they don't choose, you will choose for them. You have to be strong though and follow through on this. But it won't take long until they get on board.

So that's the '4' part of the '4 x 1'. The '1' comes from the protein section, where your children can choose between steak, chicken, fish, eggs, and so on.

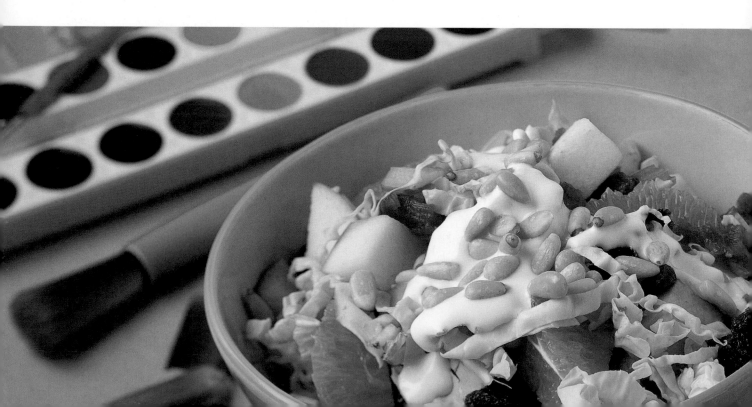

Choose Four

¼ tomato	1 radish	25g blueberries
¼ carrot	2 slices eggplant	½ pear
¼ capsicum	½ plum	½ apple
¼ onion	½ small nectarine	½ banana
2 mushrooms	¼ zucchini	½ apricot
¼ green capsicum	½ orange	1 slice of melon
mixed lettuce	½ cup cabbage	1 slice of pineapple
4 slices of cucumber	½ peach	½ mandarin
2 slices of beetroot	½ stalk celery	4 strawberries
3 medium florets broccoli	1 button squash	½ tangerine
20g mango	2 asparagus	1 kiwi fruit
	¼ grapefruit	20g peas
	2 brussels sprouts	50g pumpkin
	3 medium florets cauliflower	½ cup spinach

Choose One

80g grilled steak	100g lamb fillet
6 prawns	120g fresh white fish
50g squid	100g pork fillet
1 boiled egg	100g fresh salmon
6 oysters	
50g octopus	
120g breast chicken	

These days as soon as we walk in to the supermarket my girls know the drill and they are quick to list what they feel like. Remember, stay firm and lead by example!

This format can be used for both lunch and dinner, whether they are at school or at home.

How to get kids active!

Amy Wilkins has kindly provided helpful information in this section on keeping kids active. Amy is an award-winning music writer (APRA-AGSC Best Music for Children's Television), and business owner. Amy is a national Heart Foundation Ambassador, Juvenile Diabetes Ambassador and most recently an Australia Day Ambassador. As the co-director of Active Star Productions, Amy has produced Active Kidz Series 2 (featured on Nickelodeon) and the Active Kidz "Work It" DVD special. She has also co-produced many corporate fitness DVD's for both children and adults.

The best way to get kids active is to lead by example. You don't have to be a marathon runner, mountain climber or a gym junkie, you just need to make health and fitness a priority in your life.

The best way to do this is to make activity a natural part of your every day. For example: If you have school-age children—walk to and from school every day. If you think this is not possible because you need to drive, then think again. Park the car a good 10 minutes walk away and WALK! It is a great way to start and finish the day with your child.

Primary school-aged children are easily motivated to get active. A big part of this is playing games with their friends—so allow this to occur naturally in your day by asking kids to play at the park after school with your child. If you are inviting kids to your house for a play, encourage active games suchas tag, jumping on the trampoline, kicking and throwing balls. Be creative and imaginative— who knows, you might like to join in too.

Here are some great tips to get your kids active after school.

- Invite a friend over to play—encourage games like soccer, cricket, tip—anything to get their hearts pumping and bodies moving.

- Take your dog (or the neighbours dog) for a walk and play in the park. Take a tennis ball, frisbee or soccer ball and play with your dog—get your child to race the dog for the ball when you throw it!

- Go for a bike ride with your child or take them to the park to ride their bike. You can have races at the park and go exploring together—you never know what you may find!

- Wash the car together—a great way to keep fit and to get odd jobs done around the house.

- Grab a skipping rope and teach your child to skip. Get them to skip for as long as they can. Try to get them to skip for a little bit longer every time and beat the previous day's record. If they become an expert at this—they can try skipping backwards!

- Sign your child up for a local sports team—let them have fun meeting new people and playing a team sport.

- Set up a circuit in your back yard—set out some cones as stations and create a fun workout— you could even challenge your child and do it together!

- Take a walk to your local park and jog around the oval with your child—try timing each lap. This is a great way to monitor progress and to set challenges.

- Walk, scooter or bike ride to your local shops with your child instead of driving—this is a great way to keep fit and pick up the groceries at the same time!

- If you do not have school-age children and are in the midst of struggling with toddlers and prams— don't feel at a loss. The best way to get younger kids active is to provide them with situations that allow them to get active naturally. For example; take them to the park—let them climb, play and explore. Ask them to chase the birds/ducks/lizards. A great challenge is to tell them if they catch the bird/duck they can keep it! That will get them running for ages!

- Whatever age your children are make health and fitness a priority in your life—you will all feel the amazing benefits (not to mention sleep well).

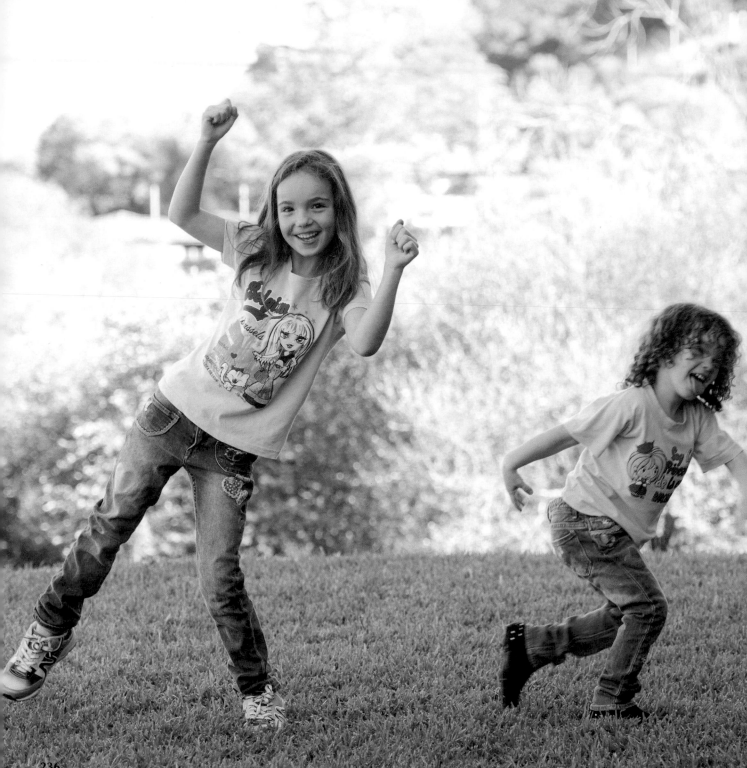

Tips from the Kids!

I asked my girls to provide some tips of their own!

Emily—5 yrs

1. Eat salad and vegetables

2. Eat fruit

3. Dance

4. Ride your bike

5. Play fun games in the playground

Jessica—8 yrs

1. Go for a run

2. Skip with a rope

3. Only eat treats sometimes

4. Play sport after school

5. Have 4 fruits or vegetables on your plate

APPENDIX

Diaries and planners

Testing Diary

Use this to complete the body composition tests (see Chapter 2) and the health and fitness tests (see Chapter 13). Redo them every 3–6 weeks. Use the space 'Other measure' to record things you may not be able to do on your own, such as blood pressure, cholesterol, blood glucose levels, body fat or use it for your own personal tests such as re-trying those pants that don't fit anymore.

Testing Diary

Use this to complete the body composition tests (see Chapter 2) and the health and fitness tests (see Chapter 13). Redo them every 3–6 weeks. Use the space 'Other measure' to record things you may not be able to do on your own, such as blood pressure, cholesterol, blood glucose levels, body fat or use it for your own personal tests such as re-trying those pants that don't fit anymore.

Test type	Test result	Re-test result
Weight		
BMI		
Resting Heart Rate		
Stomach		
Waist		
Hip		
Waist-to-hip ratio		
Timed Run/Walk	Time: RHR: WHR: Rec HR:	
Push-up test		
Abdominal test		
Sit-n-Reach test		
Other measure		
Other measure		

How to do your tests

Test type	Test description	Ideal
Weight	Take shoes and socks off. Stand on the scales with feet evenly spaced and weight evenly distributed over both feet	Compare against your own weight
BMI	Divide your weight in kilograms by your height in metres squared	20–24.9
Resting Heart Rate (RHR)	Sit down and place your first and second fingers on your carotid artery (underneath your chin on the side of your neck) or on the flipside of your wrist. Using a watch or clock to time, measure the number of times you feel it beat in 60 seconds.	< 70 bpm
Stomach	Wrap measuring tape in line with your navel	Compare against your own measurement
Waist	Measure the smallest place between your hips and your chest	<94 centimetres (37 inches) for men, < 80 centimetres (31.5 inches) for women
Hip	Take the biggest measurement at the pelvis	Compare against your own measurement

Waist-to-hip ratio	Divide your waist measurement by your hip measurement	<0.8 for women, <0.9 for men
Timed Run/ Walk	**Step 1:** Find a course that cannot be altered (so that the distance won't be different when you re-test). For example, the fence at a park or oval, between two houses or fixed points such as telegraph poles. For the best results, the test should be at least 5–8 minutes in duration. This may mean that you must walk the whole way to begin with in order to finish. **Step 2:** Measure your RHR before you warm-up. **Step 3:** Walk, run or walk/run your course and stop to measure your Working Heart Rate (WHR) at regular intervals during the test—such as every kilometre, every two to three minutes, or each time you pass a certain point. Ask a friend to write them down for you. **Step 4:** On finishing the course, record the time taken to complete the whole course. For better analysis, record times where you stopped to measure your Working Heart Rate (WHR). **Step 5:** Measure your Rec HR at the 1st, 2nd and 3rd minute after finishing. Take this as you're moving about to cool down.	Compare your results against your own score
Push-up test	Complete as many push-ups as possible in 60 seconds	Male >40, Female >30
Abdominal test	Complete as many full crunches in 20 seconds as possible	29 years old: >17, 30–39 years old: >15, 40–59 years old: >13

Sit-n-Reach test	Sit with your legs straight and feet flat up against a bench or get someone to hold them in position. Reach forward slowly, bringing your fingers toward or over your toes as far as you can. Use a tape measure or ruler and measure the gap between your hands and toes (you will need someone to help you with this). Anything before your toes is a negative reading and anything over is positive. Hold for three seconds. Do this three times and take the average.	1–7cm
Other measure:		

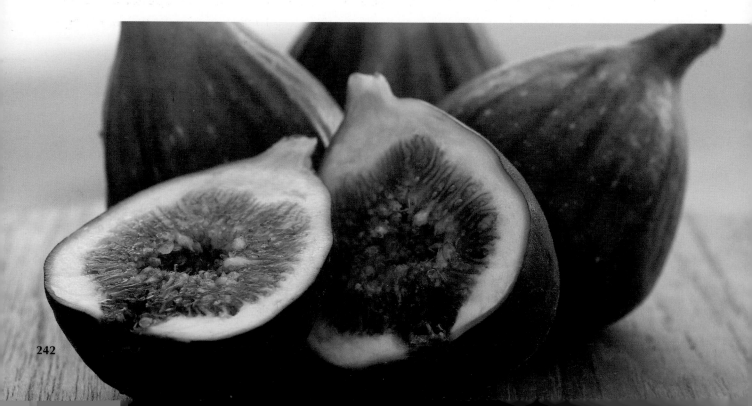

Food Diary

Use this diary to record the following:

Time: What time did I eat?

Description: What did I eat? Include specifics, because two meals that look the same can have extreme differences in their calorie content. For example, you may write down that you had a salad sandwich for lunch but did you have it with butter, cheese, or mayonnaise? These details can make a huge difference over the course of a week.

Size: Note the exact serving size.

Calories: Note the calorie amount of that food.

Daily thoughts: Use this space to record any standout moments regarding your eating behaviours around any of the meals, such as: What was I thinking/doing before I ate? What was I thinking/doing while I ate? Satisfaction/fullness on completion? Cravings? Emotions before, during and after eating? Taking notes on your eating behaviour will help you identify any emotional eating patterns and also help you identify where you might be going wrong with sticking to your diet, such as identifying a bad food choice because you were too busy or were poorly prepared.

Positive (Yourself): What positive thing have you done for yourself today (such as made a big batch of vegetable soup, stuck to my calories, cooked a new recipe, went for a walk instead of eating chocolate).
Positive (Another): What have you done for another person (such as helped the old lady down the street with her shopping, surprised your kids by taking them to the park). Keeping these daily positive notes is a way for you to see each day that you are good and you deserve this!

Water: Tick off at least eight glasses a day plus extra for exercise (one glass before your workout, one glass-worth sipped during your workout and one more glass after your workout).

Sample Food Diary

Monday:

Time	Description	Size	Calories
7am	Oats made with water	¾ cup	112
	Skim milk	½ cup	44
10am	Apple	1 medium	78
1pm	Roast beef and tomato sandwich		
	Wholemeal bread	2 thin slices	143
	Roast beef	2 thin slices	151
	Tomato	3 thin slices	8
	Banana	1 small	77
3pm	Strawberry low-fat yoghurt	200g (7¼oz)	180
7pm	Steak—grilled	200g (7¼oz)	392
	Carrot	½ cup	29
	Cauliflower	3 florets	13
	Broccoli	½ cup	27
8pm	Low-fat ice cream	2 regular scoops	158
		Total:	**1412**

Daily Thoughts: ....

Positive (Yourself): ....

Positive (Another): ....

Water: ■ ■ ■ ■ ■ ■ □ □ □ □ □

Food Diary

Time	Description	Size	Calories

Daily Thoughts: ....
Positive (Yourself): ....
Positive (Another): ....
Water: ☐☐☐☐☐☐☐☐☐☐

Activity Diary

This space logs all of your physical activity—everything from a workout to climbing the stairs, to doing the housework. Remember, it all adds up! Use this diary to record the following:

Time: What time I did the activity

Type: What the activity was

Duration: For how long?

Calories: Calories burned doing the activity

Daily calorie deficit: Add your BMR to total calories burned for the day, then subtract the total calories consumed. (See Chapter 7 and also *www.raykellyfitness.com*) For example, if your BMI is 1800 calories, and you burn 400 calories in 'activity for the day', and you consume 1200 calories in food, then your Daily Calorie Deficit would be: 1800 + 400 – 1200 = 1000 calorie deficit. (Remember, it's ideal to make at least a 500 calorie deficit to lose approximately half a kilogram or 1 pound per week.)

Sleep: Hours slept

Daily goals completed: Tick this box to confirm you achieved your Daily Process Goals: (see Chapter 6).

Daily thoughts: Use this space to record anything that affected your activity levels for the day, such as 'I had a really busy day, and struggled to exercise' or 'Felt really unmotivated to workout'. Logging these thoughts can help pick up patterns that prevent you from sticking to regular activity and exercise.

Sample Activity Diary

Day: Tuesday

Exercise

Time	Type	Duration	Calories	Goals completed
7.30	Walk along lake	60min	420	
		Total:	**420**	

Incidental Activity

Time	Type	Duration	Calories	Goals completed
12.30	Walk to deliver material to head office	20min	140	
5.30	Played with kids	30min	137	
8.00	Ironing	20min	81	
		Total:	**358**	

*Daily calorie deficit: 1800 + 420 + 358 - 1600 = 978

Sleep: ■ ■ ■ ■ ■ ■ □ □ □ □

Daily goals completed: ☑

Daily thoughts: Felt very stressed as I left for my walk as the kids were fighting but came back feeling much better. Glad I went!

* 1800 (assuming this is your BMI) + 420 (calories burned through exercise) + 358 (calories burned through incidental activity) – 1600 (assuming this is your calorie content for the day) = 978

Activity Diary

Day:

Exercise

Time	Type	Duration	Calories	Goals completed

Incidental Activity

Time	Type	Duration	Calories	Goals completed

Daily calorie deficit:

Sleep: ☐ ☐ ☐ ☐ ☐ ☐ ☐ ☐ ☐ ☐

Daily goals completed: ☐

Daily thoughts:

Calorie Cutting Planner

Use this planner to see where you can drop 500 calories (see Chapter 10).

Day:

Time	Description	Size	Calories
		Total:	

My list of 500-calorie reductions

Favourite Foods Planner

We all have favourite foods that we like to have quite regularly. To save you from continuously searching through your Calorie Counter for their values, record them here.

Food/meal	Size	Calories
	Total:	

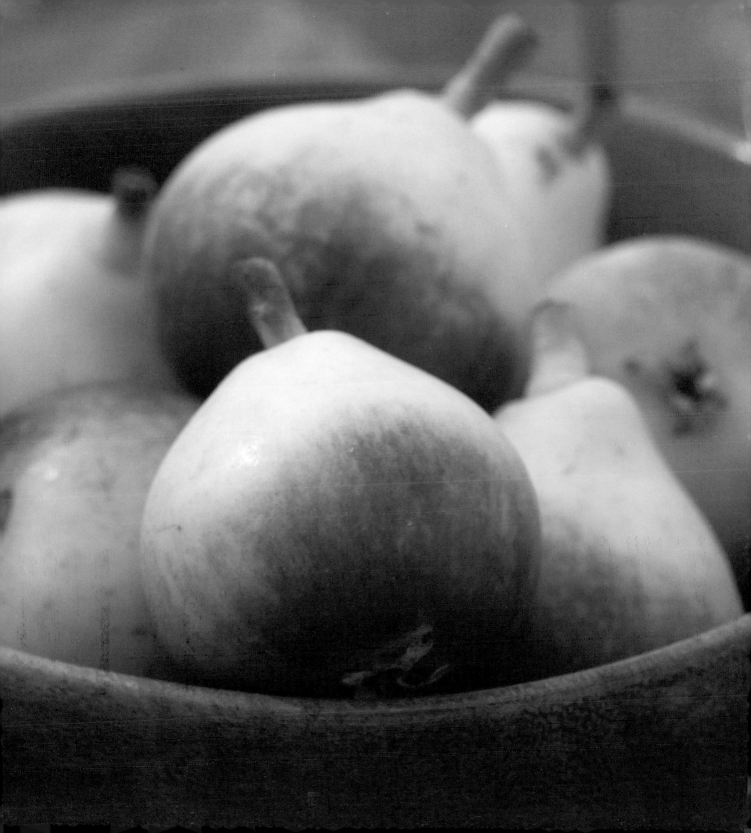

Time Management Planner

Use this planner if you constantly find yourself saying 'I don't have enough time', be it to exercise, walk to the corner shop, cook a healthy meal, go grocery shopping and so on.

- Write down the times you wake up and go to bed

- Write down the periods where you are at work or school

- Write down your meal times

Okay, so these are the necessary times taken care of. Now work in your planned exercise, activity and healthy-things-to-do periods for each day. Remember, if you can't find a good 30–60 minute block to exercise, then find two shorter workout periods. Or, factor in even more incidental activity.

Time	Monday	Tuesday	Wednesday	Thursday	Friday	Saturday	Sunday
5							
6							
7							
8							
9							
10							
11							
12							
1							
2							
3							
4							
5							
6							
7							
8							
9							
10							
11							

Pay-it-Forward Planner

Use this planner to factor in extra calories you want to consume at upcoming special occasions and work out how you will burn the calories four weeks in advance (see Chapter 18). For example: If you walk briskly (4 METS) for 60 minutes each day and want to factor in treats totalling 1800 calories, you would need to share the extra 1800 calories over 28 days (4 weeks). This means you have to burn an extra 72 calories in each session. If you're 100 kilograms, for example, you'll need to walk 11 minutes extra each session. The pay-it-back section allows you to burn it off after the event in case you didn't stick to your plan to burn it in advance.

Sample Pay-it-Forward Planner

Special occasion: Christmas Lunch

Date: 25/12/08

Treat of choice	Size	Calories
½ bottle wine	375ml	280
Turkey roast with skin	100g	170
2 roast potatoes	200g	250
Slice Christmas cake with icing	80g	320
	Total:	1020

	Extra exercise	Calories
Pay-it-forward Week 1	Extra 3 minutes* of running each day	36.75
Pay-it-forward Week 2	Extra 3 minutes of running each day	36.75
Pay-it-forward Week 3	Extra 3 minutes of running each day	36.75
Pay-it-forward Week 4	Extra 3 minutes of running each day	36.75

Pay-it-back	-	
	Total:	1029

*Based on 70-kilogram person

Pay-it-Forward Planner

Special occasion:

Date:

Treat of choice	Size	Calories
	Total:	

	Extra exercise	Calories
Pay-it-forward Week 1		
Pay-it-forward Week 2		
Pay-it-forward Week 3		
Pay-it-forward Week 4		
Pay-it-back		
	Total:	

US $18.99

UK £12.99